AF228886

Screen Addiction:
A Teen Epidemic

Bradley Steffens

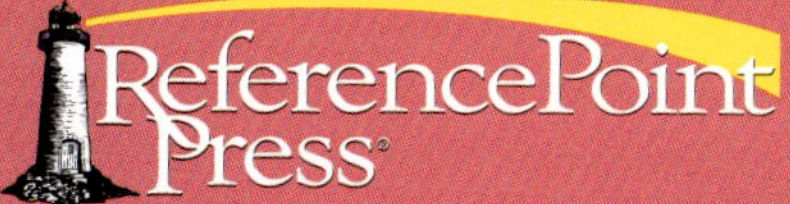

San Diego, CA

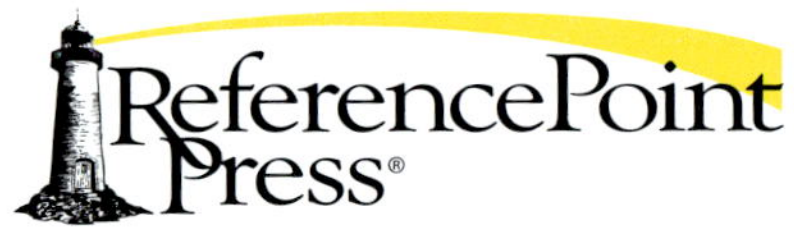

About the Author

Bradley Steffens is a novelist, poet, and award-winning author of more than sixty nonfiction books for children and young adults.

Picture Credits:

Cover: Leszek Czerwonka/Shutterstock Images
 6: FrimuFilms/Shutterstock
10: insta_photos/Shutterstock
13: FangXiaNuo/iStock
17: BAZA Production/Shutterstock
21: Syda Productions/Shutterstock
24: Rohane Hamilton/Shutterstock
27: VALUA VITALY/Shutterstock
31: Monkey Business Images/Shutterstock
33: tommaso79/Shutterstock
36: VH-studio/Shutterstock
40: Gorodenkoff/Shutterstock
43: Joshua Resnick/Shutterstock
48: Just Life/Shutterstock
49: Wachiwit/Shutterstock
54: SDI Productions/iStock

LIBRARY OF CONGRESS CATALOGING-IN-PUBLICATION DATA

Names: Steffens, Bradley, 1955- author.
Title: Screen addiction : a teen epidemic / by Bradley Steffens.
Description: San Diego, CA : ReferencePoint Press, 2023. | Includes bibliographical references and index.
Identifiers: LCCN 2022010963 (print) | LCCN 2022010964 (ebook) | ISBN 9781678203528 (library binding) | ISBN 9781678203535 (ebook)
Subjects: LCSH: Internet addiction--Juvenile literature.
Classification: LCC RC569.5.I54 S744 2023 (print) | LCC RC569.5.I54 (ebook) | DDC 616.85/84--dc23/eng/20220318
LC record available at https://lccn.loc.gov/2022010963
LC ebook record available at https://lccn.loc.gov/2022010964

A Growing Crisis

In February 2020, a college student named Lev described how his once-harmless hobby of watching movies was taking over his life:

> I watch movies on my laptop for hours on end. It takes up all my study time, and before I know it the semester is over and another begins and I'm almost failing all units. I just feel like time is rushing and nothing is happening in my life except fantasizing what I see in movies (healthy relationships, vacations, a lot of friends, creativity, making an impact in the world . . .).

> I currently feel so empty and have none of those. It has become my hideout from life. I feel alone, I don't interact with people a lot and this has taken away almost all my self esteem, ability to communicate with people and all of my social life. I have these big plans and ideas in my mind but always get carried away by movies looking for a "high point" and filling a void which never gets filled.

> Under the current coronavirus crisis schools have been closed and I find myself watching up to 20 hours a day even struggling to get time to sleep or cook for myself. I feel that I finally need to have a control of my life again and become a better person.[1]

Although Lev's situation is extreme, his increased use of electronic media during the pandemic is not unique. In November 2021, researchers at the University of California, San Francisco, reported that the amount of time teenagers spent in front of screens for non-school-related purposes—including gaming, texting, video chatting, browsing the internet, interacting with social media, and watching movies, videos, or television shows—had more than doubled during the pandemic, from 3.8 to 7.7 hours per day.

The Potential Harms of Digital Dependence

Mental health professionals found the sudden increase in screen time alarming because it was accompanied by increases in the number of teens reporting anxiety, depression, and suicidal thinking. The amount of time that teens were spending with their electronic devices was so concerning that the US surgeon general, Vivek H. Murthy, discussed it when he issued a formal advisory in December 2021 alerting the medical community to a mental health crisis among America's youth. "Digital technologies can expose children to bullying, contribute to obesity and eating disorders, trade off with sleep, encourage children to negatively compare themselves to others, and lead to depression, anxiety, and self-harm," stated the surgeon general's report. "Technology companies must step up and take responsibility for creating a safe digital environment for children and youth."[2]

For teens like Lev, large amounts of time spent in front of a screen can morph into an addiction to electronic devices and the activities they make possible. A 2020 study by Oxford University found that half of all teen and young adult cell phone users say they feel addicted to their devices. The World Health Organization (WHO), an agency of the United Nations that is concerned with global

"Digital technologies can expose children to bullying, contribute to obesity and eating disorders, trade off with sleep, encourage children to negatively compare themselves to others, and lead to depression, anxiety, and self-harm."[2]

—Vivek H. Murthy, US surgeon general

public health, estimates that 3 to 4 percent of gamers worldwide are addicted to playing video games, including 5 million in the United States alone. And a study by researchers at the University of Michigan–Flint found that 6 percent of social media users—about 9 million Americans—are addicted to social media.

Toward Screen Addiction

The types of addictions described by Oxford University, the WHO, and the University of Michigan–Flint—often grouped together with video and movie watching under the umbrella term *screen addiction*—are known as behavioral addictions. A behavioral addiction is a mental health condition in which an individual engages in a particular behavior and is unable to stop engaging in it, even if the behavior causes the person harm.

The key components of behavioral addiction have been described by Mark D. Griffiths, a professor at Nottingham Trent Uni-

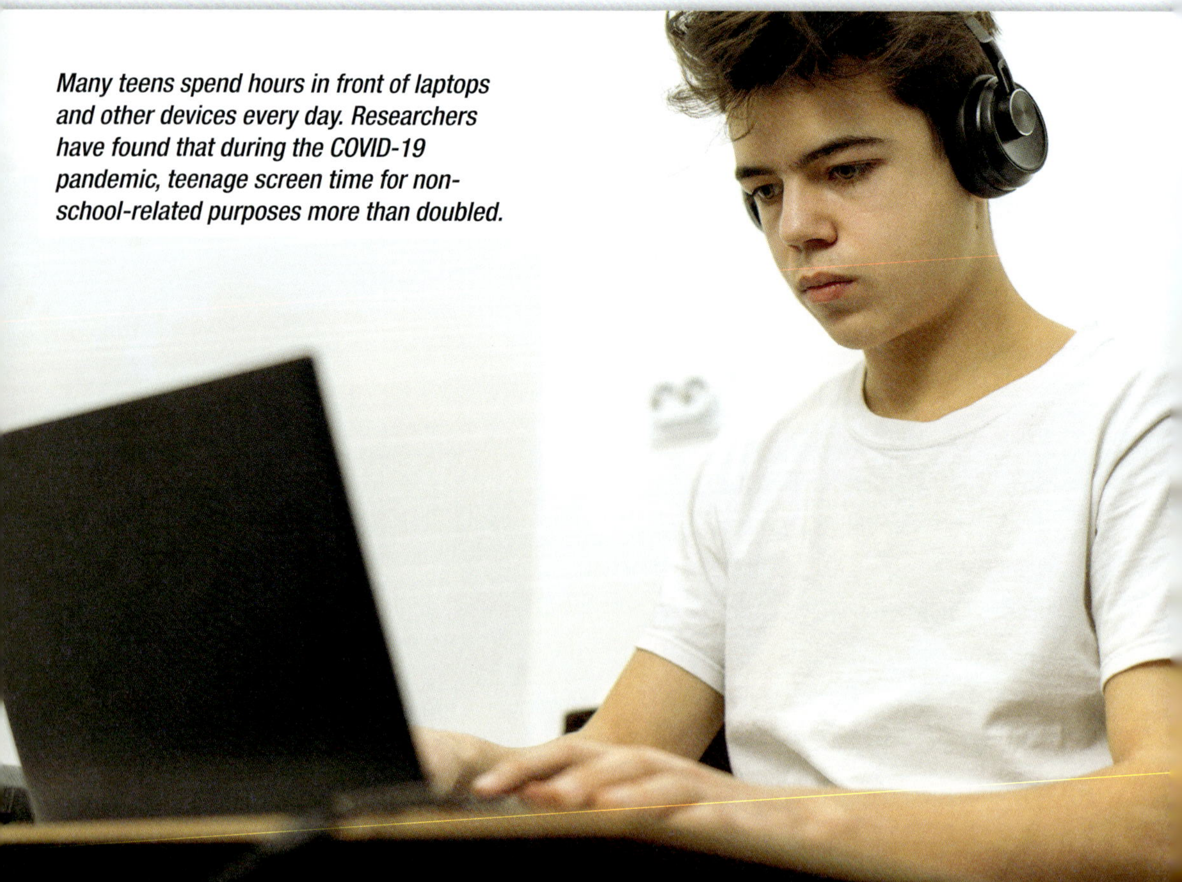

Many teens spend hours in front of laptops and other devices every day. Researchers have found that during the COVID-19 pandemic, teenage screen time for non-school-related purposes more than doubled.

versity in England and one of the first psychologists to publish research recognizing screen addiction. Griffiths defines a behavioral addiction as an activity engaged in so excessively that it damages personal, family, or professional life. He lists six hallmarks of behavioral addiction: 1) salience, when a behavior becomes a most important part of a person's life; 2) mood modification, when a person uses a behavior to alter his or her moods or escape from problems; 3) tolerance, when a person has to spend more time engaged in a behavior to produce the same feelings of well-being; 4) withdrawal symptoms, when a person has unpleasant feelings or physical sensations when not able to engage in a behavior; 5) conflict, when a behavior creates relationship problems or disrupts everyday life; and 6) relapse, when a person tries to limit or end a behavior but reverts to excessive use. Any behavior that meets these six criteria is an addiction, Griffiths says.

Some behavioral addictions, including gambling disorder and shopping addiction, have been formally recognized by the medical community. However, since the overuse of technological devices is a new phenomenon, its addictive properties are still being studied. Nevertheless, members of the mental health community are already applying time-tested addiction treatments to people whose lives are out of control because of their involvement with electronic devices.

The Fear of Missing Out

"When I was 14, I got an LG Optimus smartphone, passed on from a school friend. It had a touchscreen and felt like it was from the future," remembers Moya Lothian-McLean, an editor with the online British magazine *gal-dem*. "No longer could my mum boot me off the computer. . . . I could talk with my friends into the wee hours, refreshing the Facebook browser page every minute to see if their latest missive had come through. Never had I felt so alive. At the time, the entire world was at my fingertips, anytime, any place." Now, however, Lothian-McLean realizes that she cannot control her use of electronic devices. She continuously switches between screens, unable to focus on her work:

> I find myself reaching for my phone every few minutes, snatching it up when I get stuck on a sentence I'm typing and need to "reset" my mind by blankly scrolling. Sometimes Twitter will be open on a laptop screen in front of me and I'll find myself idly pulling up the little blue bird app on my phone too. A great feeling of distress runs through me when I cannot spot my phone where I think I left it.[3]

A Basic Need

Lothian-McLean's screen activity is not driven by curiosity or any rational motive. It is a compulsion, fueled by anxiety. She has a deep-seated concern that she might be unaware of something happening on her phone or on social media. Screen addiction experts call this anxiety the fear of missing out, or FOMO.

FOMO was first defined by researchers at the University of Essex in England as "the uneasy and sometimes all-consuming feeling that you're missing out—that your peers are doing, in the know about, or in possession of more or something better than you."[4] Since social media gives the user a real-time or near-real-time window into the activities of others, people today are much more aware of what their peers are doing. As a result, concerns about being out of touch or left behind are greater today than in the past.

The feelings are especially intense for teens, who have a deep need to fit in with their peers. Amy Summerville, a professor of psychology at Miami University in Ohio, points out that such feelings are not superficial. FOMO is an extension of the biological need for socialization and inclusion. Once basic needs such as food, shelter, and water are met, inclusion and social interaction are high on the list of human needs.

A Source of Anxiety

Because the need for social acceptance is so deep, FOMO can be strong and persistent, creating a mental health condition known as anxiety. To alleviate this anxiety, people in the grips of FOMO will check their devices. According to a Pew Research study, 45 percent of teens say that they spend hours online each day, with most of that time spent checking social media. They do so not out of genuine curiosity about their friends' activities but rather to soothe their emotions. Engaging in an activity to modify a mood is a classic symptom of a behavioral addiction. "You let it go from being something you enjoy to something that's controlling you,"[5] says Douglas A. Gentile, a professor of psychology at Iowa State University.

Unfortunately, checking a device provides only temporary relief from the anxiety, and over time the behavior makes the anxiety worse. Social media users instinctively know that as soon as they leave the website, someone could post new content. As a result, FOMO returns almost as soon as users leave the site. And because they have just checked their accounts, the awareness of what might be going on in social media remains at the top of their minds, fueling the urge to check their devices again. The never-ending cycle adds up to an astonishing level of involvement with screens. According to a study conducted by dscout, a technology research firm, cell phone users tap,

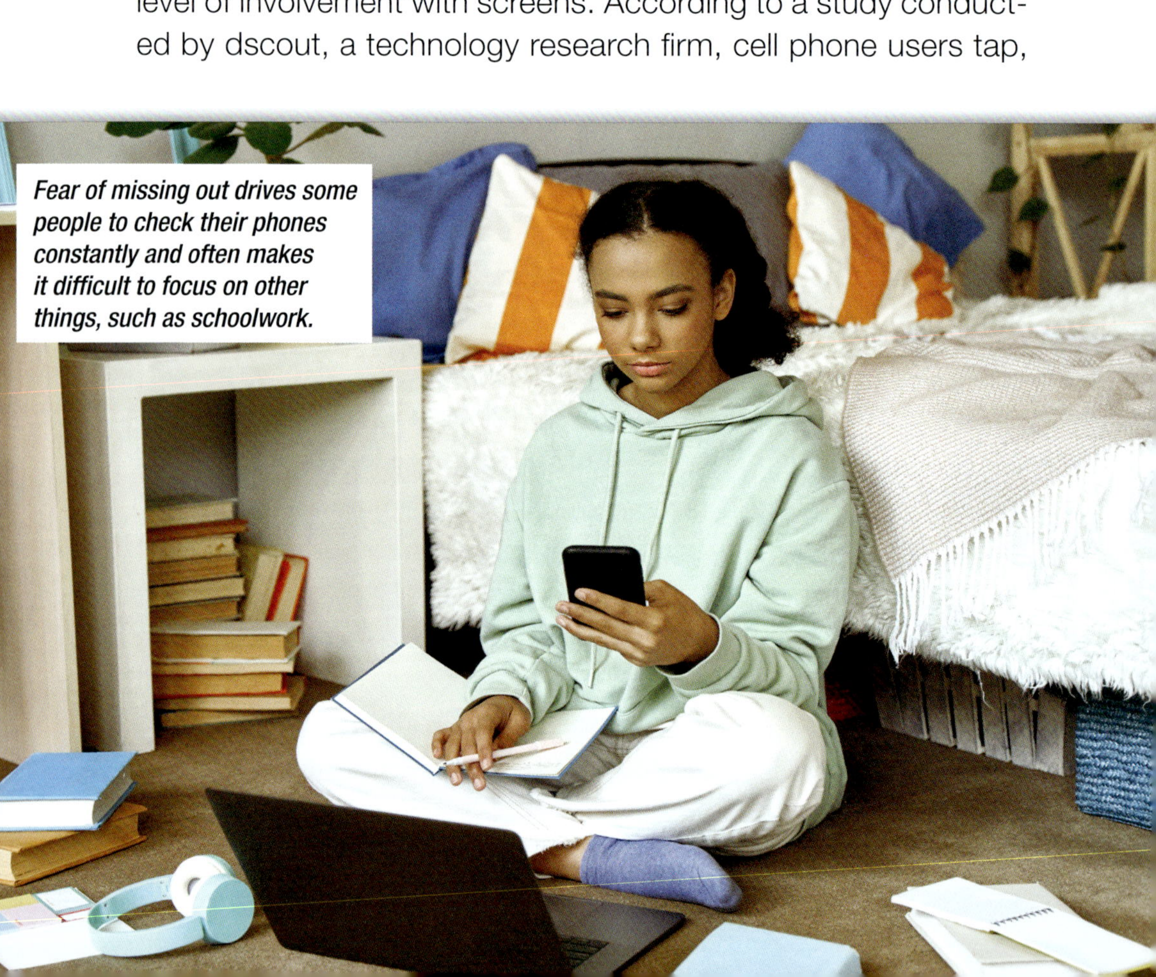

Fear of missing out drives some people to check their phones constantly and often makes it difficult to focus on other things, such as schoolwork.

scroll, or swipe their screens an average of 2,617 times a day to check on social media updates, read messages, and perform other tasks.

Disconnecting from the Real World

One of the problems with the continual checking of devices is that it prevents users from being aware of and involved with things around them. This disconnection with real life and real relationships does not relieve the user's anxiety. It heightens it. "When an individual is not engaging in the world in a healthy way—interacting with others, managing themselves in challenging situations, whether it's in classes or speaking up in class, going on interviews, dealing with conflict with peers—and instead increase[s] their online presence, this can exacerbate their feelings of alienation, hopelessness, isolation, anxiety, and depression,"[6] says Anne Marie Albano, director of the Columbia University Clinic for Anxiety and Related Disorders.

Albano's analysis is based on multiple studies showing that those most at risk for anxiety and depression often turn to screens to modify their moods. In 2021, Common Sense Media, a nonprofit organization that studies media and technology, reported that young people with depressive symptoms are nearly twice as likely as those without depression to say they use social media almost constantly (34 percent versus 18 percent).

The same study found that 43 percent of fourteen- to twenty-two-year-old social media users said that using social media when they are depressed, stressed, or anxious usually makes them feel better, but nearly one in five—17 percent—said that engaging in social media at such times made them feel worse.

FOMO Marketing

Recently, marketers have realized that FOMO can be used to manipulate consumers into making impulsive buying decisions. Marketing consultant Steve Hogan describes this technique, known as FOMO marketing:

> In case you're allergic to social media and haven't ever before heard the term, FOMO means "the fear of missing out." . . . FOMO marketing refers to messaging that appeals to consumers' desire to latch on to every opportunity before it slips through their fingers. Many people would rather make an impulse purchase than regret failing to act later. . . .
>
> Language matters a lot when it comes to FOMO marketing. You want your audience to feel as though time is running out and that they're about to lose on an amazing offer.
>
> When you're crafting your marketing materials, use strong verbs and adjectives to instill FOMO in your target audience. Phrases like "don't miss this" and "while supplies last" are good examples, but you can get more creative.
>
> FOMO marketing is real. So is FOMO itself. If you create a situation in which your audience has to act fast to get an opportunity they might not get again, you'll encourage sales and conversions.

Steve Hogan, "10 Effective FOMO Marketing Techniques to Increase Online Results," *Daily Egg* (blog), Crazy Egg, July 26, 2021. www.crazyegg.com.

"For those who have severe depression, social media plays an outsized role—more important for inspiration, support, and connection, but also more likely to make respondents more anxious, lonely, and depressed."[7]

Internal research conducted by Facebook and leaked to the public in September 2021 came to the same conclusion. The Facebook researchers found that 31 percent of teens with mental health issues said that browsing through photos on the photo-sharing app Instagram, which is owned by Facebook, worsened their mental health. Nevertheless, the vulnerable teens continued to expose themselves to the content because of FOMO.

"Young people are acutely aware that Instagram can be bad for their mental health," wrote the researchers, "yet are compelled to spend time on the app for fear of missing out on cultural and social trends."[8]

Surprising Effects of Family Structure

Although the negative effects of FOMO are greatest among teens with mental health issues, it appears that other factors that generally improve mental health did not make teens immune from FOMO. For example, a 2020 study by researchers at the Centre for Sociological Research in Belgium found that adolescents from intact families—those in which both parents are present— had higher rates of FOMO than did adolescents in nonintact families. "This finding was not in line with our first hypothesis, in which we expected that adolescents from intact families experience less FOMO than adolescents from non-intact families,"[9] the researchers admitted.

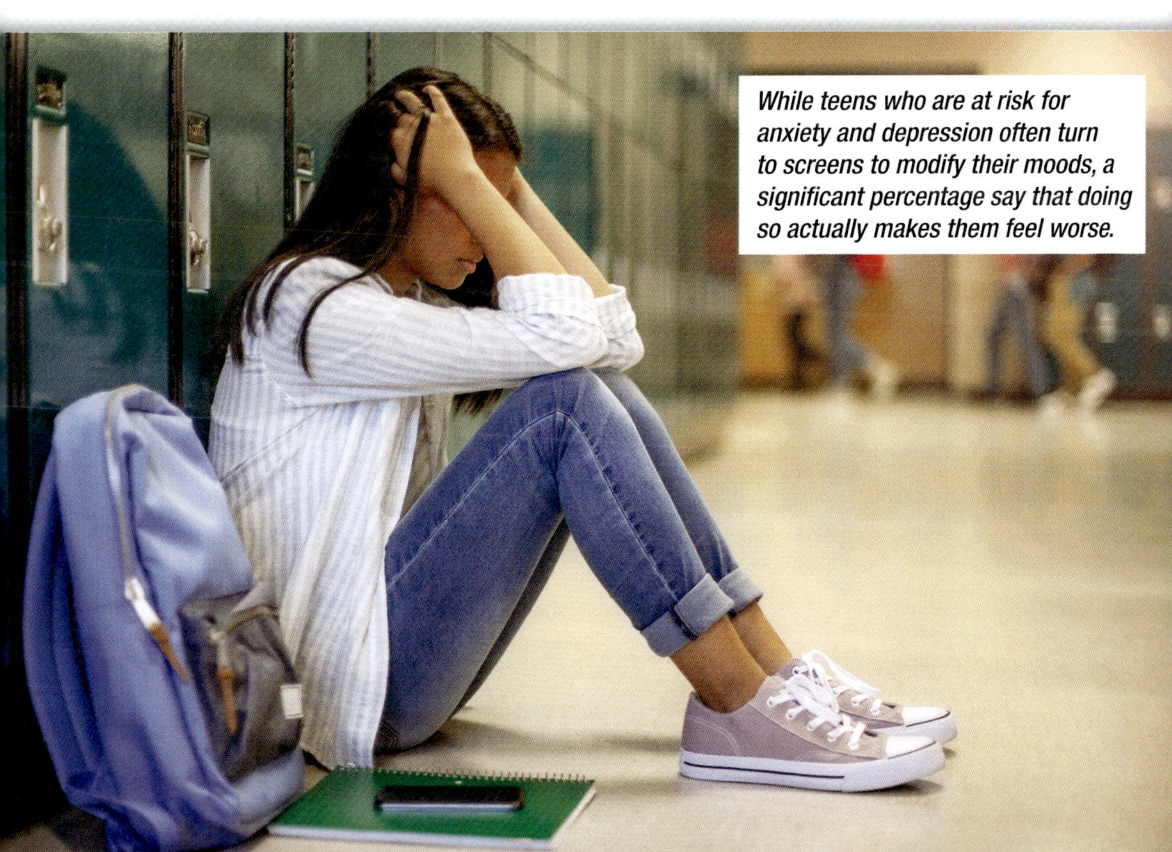

While teens who are at risk for anxiety and depression often turn to screens to modify their moods, a significant percentage say that doing so actually makes them feel worse.

FOMO and Pedestrian Risks

Teens and children in the throes of FOMO are a danger to themselves as pedestrians. A 2020 study by researchers at Canada's University of Calgary found that one in five high schoolers and one in eight middle schoolers were distracted when crossing streets in school zones. Of the distractions, the vast majority—80 percent—involved electronic devices. Only 20 percent were due to talking to other students. "As expected, texting or browsing had the most detrimental effects on hits and close calls and looking left and right," stated the researchers. "Texting requires a pedestrian to repeatedly divert their eyes away from the walking environment and traffic, towards the screen of the phone, to type and read messages. Browsing requires repeated device interactions and information scanning. If pedestrians do not look left and right when crossing a street, detection of vehicles likely also decreases."

Sarah M. Simmons et al., "Plight of the Distracted Pedestrian: A Research Synthesis and Meta-Analysis of Mobile Phone Use on Crossing Behaviour," *Injury Prevention*, April 2020. https://injury prevention.bmj.com.

The researchers knew that adolescents from nonintact families use social media more often than adolescents from intact families do. Since their own study showed that higher social media use is a risk factor of FOMO, the researchers assumed that adolescents from nonintact families should experience more FOMO, but this was not the case. They explained this surprising result by drawing on other research, which has found that teens in nonintact families tend to develop personal independence sooner than teens in intact families. "Studies have shown that adolescents from non-intact families report higher feelings of independence than adolescents from intact families: adolescents from non-intact families often face additional household tasks and caretaking responsibilities for younger siblings and are thus likely to become more independent at an earlier age," wrote the researchers. "While some studies have found that these role shifts are detrimental to adolescents, others found that adolescents from non-intact families understand the necessity of increasing self-reliance and enjoy the benefits of greater independence and decision making."[10] As a result of their independence, teens from non-intact families are less reliant on social media and other screen activities for feelings of socialization, inclusion, and self-esteem.

Another surprising result from the 2020 study was that teens with strong relationships with their fathers experienced less FOMO than those with strong relationships with their mothers. "Curiously enough, and contrary to much of the literature, the association of the relationship with the father with [lower] FOMO is stronger than the association with the relationship with the mother." Again, the researchers turned to other research to explain this surprising result:

> There is some evidence that relationships with fathers may be taken less "for granted" by adolescents than those with mothers, and that "high quality, positive relationships with fathers [are] indicative of individual competence and desirability in relationships. . . ." Relationships with mothers, in contrast, are perhaps viewed as "granted" or expected, such that individual performance or competency in the relationship is of less influence on levels of anxiety or FOMO.[11]

Distracted Driving

Mental health problems are not the only risks posed by FOMO. It also plays a role in the soaring numbers of distraction-related traffic accidents, pedestrian accidents, and accidental falls. According to the National Highway Traffic Safety Administration (NHTSA), an agency of the federal government, in fatal traffic accidents in 2019, drivers aged fifteen to nineteen years old were more likely to be distracted than drivers aged twenty and older. In at least 8 percent of the fatal crashes, drivers aged fifteen to nineteen were distracted at the time of the crash.

Although drivers can be distracted by many things, most distractions involve electronic devices. According to Cambridge Mobile Telematics (CMT), a software company specializing in safe driving apps, engaging with electronic screens makes up more than two-thirds (68 percent) of all driving distractions, with eating (10 percent) and talking to other people (22 percent) making up the remaining third. "Multiple surveys of drivers conducted by CMT asking about their behavior confirm they are mostly distracted by their phones," states the company's 2020 report, *The Harsh Realities of Phone Distraction*. "It is the source of the calls, texts, videos, navigation, and social connection that the majority fall victim to on a regular basis."[12]

Interacting with social media is particularly dangerous because of the phenomenon known as the "distraction hangover." When a driver is distracted, it is for an average of twenty-three seconds. During this time, a vehicle can travel the length of more than five football fields at speeds above 40 miles per hour (64 kmh). Part of the twenty-three seconds is the distraction hangover—the continued impact of distraction after the actual event has ended. Based on feedback from CMT's software loaded onto thousands of drivers' phones, screen interactions such as texting, scrolling, and swiping generate "a very intense distraction hangover,"[13] increasing the risk of a hard braking event by 82 percent ten seconds after the screen interaction ends. This compares to just a 40 percent increased risk of a hard-braking event for distractions caused by moving a phone and a 60 percent increased risk from receiving a phone call.

According to the NHTSA, teens are much more likely to engage with screens while driving than any other age group. In 2020, 4.3 percent of drivers aged sixteen to twenty-four were visibly manipulating handheld devices as they drove. That compares to just 2.8 percent of drivers aged twenty-five to sixty-nine, and only 0.5 percent of drivers aged seventy and older. The number of teens engaging with screens while driving has increased by 79 percent since 2013, from 2.9 percent to 4.3 percent. Sur-

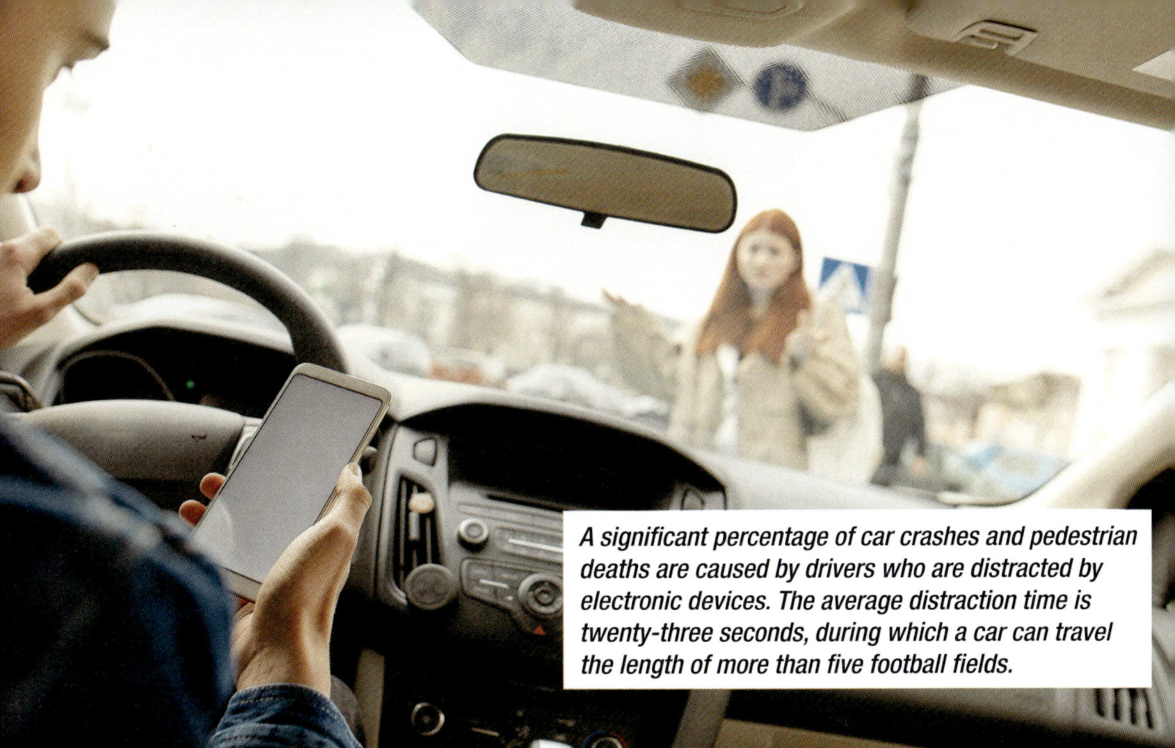

A significant percentage of car crashes and pedestrian deaths are caused by drivers who are distracted by electronic devices. The average distraction time is twenty-three seconds, during which a car can travel the length of more than five football fields.

prisingly, the increase in screen use while driving has occurred even while teens were becoming more careful about talking on cell phones while driving. According to the NHTSA, the number of teens speaking while holding a cell phone has decreased 56 percent since 2013, from 5.9 percent to just 2.6 percent.

No Safe Space

Screen distractions also play a role in accidents causing the deaths of pedestrians. The Governors Highway Safety Association (GHSA) reported in 2021 that the rate of pedestrian deaths increased more than 20 percent in the first half of 2020 despite the number of vehicle miles traveled having decreased by 16.5 percent due to the COVID-19 pandemic. One reason for the increase was that, with fewer cars on the road, average vehicle speeds rose. But another factor was an increase in distracted driving due to screen overuse. "Walking should not be a life and death undertaking, yet many factors have combined to put pedestrians at historic levels of risk,"[14] comments Jonathan Adkins, executive director of the GHSA. "We are crazy distracted," says

Melody Geraci, deputy executive director of the Active Transportation Alliance, a Chicago nonprofit organization dedicated to transportation safety. "After speeding and the failure to yield, distractions are the number three cause [of pedestrian fatalities], particularly by electronic devices."[15]

FOMO is also behind dangerous accidents in the home. "Before I bought an iPhone, I took baths and showers with my tablet, and it was not waterproof," says Tracey Folly, a columnist and blogger. "That's how terrified I was that I would miss something. FOMO is real."[16] In December 2021, a thirteen-year-old girl in Mâcon, France, died after accidentally dropping her cell phone into her bath while the phone was plugged into a charger. The teen's grieving mother spoke out about cell phone overuse: "This must be a warning to other teenagers, because they all have their phones implanted in their hands, so to speak."[17]

According to Pew Research, 95 percent of US teens have access to a cell phone, and nearly half say they are almost always on the internet. Much of this activity is due to a fear of missing out. The drive to engage with their screens is so strong that many teens put themselves and others in danger, mentally and physically. The fact that they persist in the behavior suggests that in many cases they are on the verge of screen addiction or are already there.

CHAPTER TWO

The Risks of Social Media

On October 3, 2021, former Facebook employee Frances Haugen dropped a bombshell on the world of social media. In an interview with the CBS prime-time news magazine *60 Minutes*, Haugen told reporter Scott Pelley and the millions of Americans who had tuned in to the program that researchers at Facebook, which owns the photo-sharing app Instagram, had found that Instagram software and content posed dangers to teenagers, especially teen girls. Interviews with thousands of Instagram users found that two-thirds of teen girls had bad feelings about comparisons they made between themselves and others on the app, with half of them saying that their negative social comparisons were about beauty and weight. About a third (32 percent) of teen girls said that when they felt bad about their bodies, Instagram made them feel worse. "Comparisons on Instagram can change how young women view and describe themselves,"[18] warned the researchers.

Feeding the Urge to Lose Weight

Struggles with body image can cause some teen girls to develop an obsessive desire to lose weight, and that can lead to an eating disorder such as anorexia or bulimia. "I keep looking at these images . . . sometimes I just don't eat or try to eat less,"[19] said one teen girl interviewed by the Facebook researchers. Worse, Instagram's software works in such a way that if a teen shows an interest in posts about fasting, skipping meals, and even purging through self-induced vomiting, the software will automatically serve up even more posts on these topics as a way of keeping the user engaged with the app. "The algorithms will say, 'Ooh, people engage with this topic the most. Let's show it to you more,'" explained Haugen. "And that's part of the danger for like teenagers, right? Part of the reason why these teen girls are getting eating disorders is they one time look up weight loss and the algorithm's like, 'Oh great. We'll keep showing you more and more extreme weight loss things.'"[20]

Not surprisingly, repeated exposure to such posts can affect the thoughts and emotions of some teen users. This is what happened to a fifteen-year-old Connecticut teen. Her mother emailed her senator, Richard Blumenthal, when she heard Haugen testifying before Congress after going public with Facebook's research. The mother said she was in tears as she listened to Haugen describe how Facebook's algorithms exposed at-risk teens to potentially damaging images:

My 15-year-old daughter loved her body—and at 14 was on Instagram constantly, and maybe posting too much. Suddenly, she started hating her body. With her body dysmorphia [a mental disorder involving obsessive focus on a perceived flaw in appearance], and now anorexia, she was in deep, deep trouble before we found treatment. I fear [she'll] never be the same. I am broken hearted.[21]

According to the Facebook researchers, 17 percent of teen girls said Instagram worsened eating disorders. "And what's super tragic is Facebook's own research says, as these young women begin to consume this—this eating disorder content, they get more and more depressed," explained Haugen. "And it actually makes them use the app more. And so, they end up in this feedback cycle where they hate their bodies more and more."[22]

From Inspired User to Self-Hating Influencer

Anastasia Vlasova, an eighteen-year-old from Reston, Virginia, is one of those teens who got caught up in a negative feedback cycle. She opened her Instagram account when she was thirteen and was fascinated by what she saw. "When I went on Instagram, all I saw were images of chiseled bodies, perfect abs and women doing 100 burpees in 10 minutes,"[23] says Vlasova. At first, she felt inspired by the images. She tried to eat better and work out so she could look more like her idols on Instagram. Within a few months, she opened her own fitness account and began to build a following on Instagram.

Vlasova's success made her want even more followers. Soon, Instagram was at the center of her life, pushing aside her other interests. "Everything became incredibly Instagram-centric because

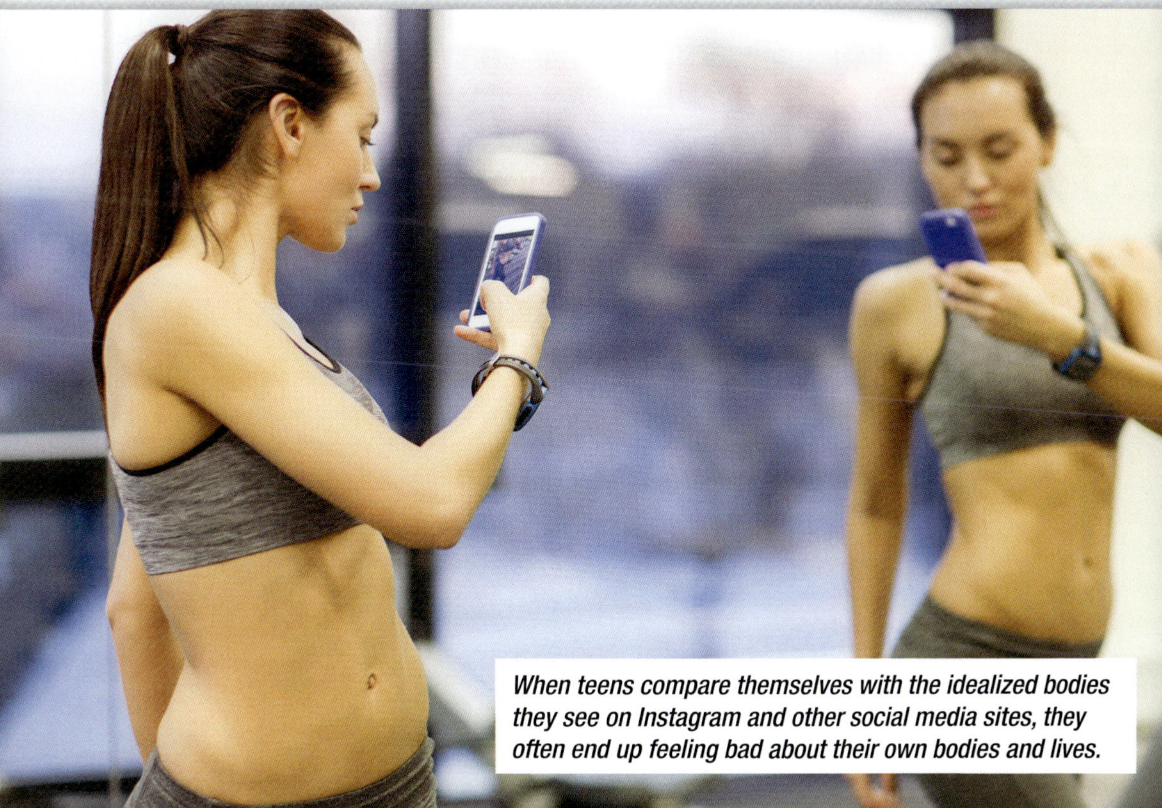

When teens compare themselves with the idealized bodies they see on Instagram and other social media sites, they often end up feeling bad about their own bodies and lives.

I was super focused on expanding my account as much as possible," she says. She began to check her Instagram account around the clock. "I remember during school I would take bathroom breaks and when I would go into the stall . . . I would go on my phone and I would be on Instagram liking people's posts, making sure that I didn't miss a single one from the past hour while I was in class."[24]

Vlasova found that the more followers she had, the more pressure she put on herself to look good. She would look at other fitness influencers to get inspired, but instead she would end up comparing herself to them and feeling worse about herself. She went from eating well to starving herself before photo shoots and bingeing afterward. "I definitely realized that a lot of the content that was produced by some of my favorite fitness influencers triggered my binges or my restrictive cycles,"[25] she said. She punished herself whenever she ate something she felt was unhealthy.

By eleventh grade, Vlasova's eating disorder and screen addiction were affecting every part of her life. She began to have anxiety attacks and trouble sleeping. She realized that she had all the symptoms of depression, and she began to see a counselor. During one session, she told her counselor she was having suicidal thoughts. "I told her I don't want to be here anymore, I hate myself. I hate how much I have disconnected from my friends and just from who I truly am because of the stupid eating disorder and my depression and my anxiety, and I don't know what to do."[26]

By opening up, Vlasova was able to get the help she needed. She started seeing a therapist, and she left Instagram. While feeling better herself, she sympathizes with those who are still trapped by their constant comparisons to others. "I had to live with my eating disorder for five years," she says, "and people on Instagram are still suffering."[27]

—Anastasia Vlasova, a former Instagram user

The Reality Behind the Image

Worried about the comparisons her social media followers might be making to her public image, one Instagram influencer came forward to tell the truth about her photos. Essena O'Neill, an eighteen-year-old Australian model with more than 770,000 followers on her social media channels, deleted more than two thousand of her photos from Instagram and edited her captions to expose the harsh reality behind the idealized images. O'Neill wrote:

> Not real life. Only reason we went to the beach this morning was to shoot these bikinis because the company paid me and also I looked good to society's current standards. I was born and won the genetic lottery. Why else would I have uploaded this photo? Read between the lines, or ask yourself "why does someone post a photo. . . . What is the outcome for them? To make a change? Look hot? Sell something?" I thought I was helping young girls get fit and healthy. But I only realised at 19 that placing any amount of self worth on your physical form is so limiting! I could have been writing, exploring, playing, anything beautiful and real. . . . Not trying to validate my worth through a bikini shot with no substance.

Quoted in Kim Fergusson, "A Blog Response to Essena O'Neill," *Fashion Weekly*, December 19, 2021. https://fashionweeklymag.com.

Designed for Comparison

The pressure to look good can be even worse for Black teens, says Shevon Jones, a social worker in Atlanta, Georgia. Jones observes that other Instagram users often think that Black teens look older than they really are, and they are more apt to be critical based on this misperception. "What girls often see on social media . . . can lead them to have body image issues," says Jones. "It's a very critical time and they are trying to figure out themselves and everything around them."[28]

The pressure of comparison is worse on Instagram than on other social media platforms, according to Haugen. "Facebook's

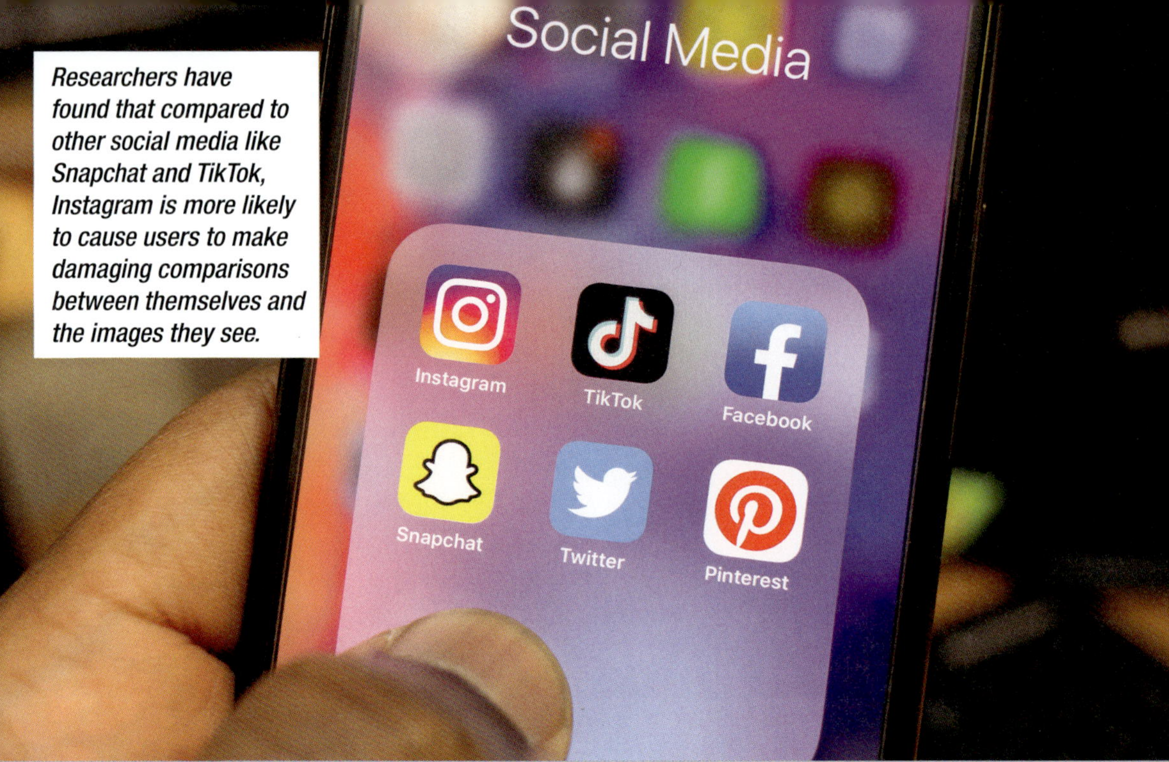

Researchers have found that compared to other social media like Snapchat and TikTok, Instagram is more likely to cause users to make damaging comparisons between themselves and the images they see.

own research says it is not just that Instagram is dangerous for teenagers, that it harms teenagers, it's that it is distinctly worse than other forms of social media,"[29] she says. By other forms of social media, Haugen is referring mainly to rival photo- and video-sharing apps, Snapchat and TikTok. The software for these apps operates differently than Instagram's does, making them less likely to invite damaging comparisons. Snapchat offers users photographic filters that alter facial images in funny ways. For example, one filter turns the user's face into a cartoon that resembles a Disney character. By doing so, Snapchat keeps the focus of its users mainly on the face. TikTok also offers funny filters for the videos its users post, including a similar Disney character filter and another that changes the user into an anime character. These and other filters distract users from comparing their bodies to those of other users. Like Instagram, TikTok serves up content to its users, but it does so not based on the interests or growing obsessions of its users but rather on which videos are most popular at the time. As a result, users are exposed to a wide range of videos rather than ones that encourage comparisons. "TikTok is about doing fun things with your friends,

Snapchat is about faces and augmented reality," says Haugen. "But Instagram is about bodies, and about comparing lifestyles."[30]

The comparisons some Instagram users make can cause them to feel inferior to the other people they see on Instagram. But what many Instagram users, including teens, do not realize is that they are not comparing themselves to "normal" Instagram users. They often are seeing models who are paid by companies to promote their products. Known as Instagram influencers, or social media influencers, these models do not take their own photos, even when they appear to be selfies. Instead, their pictures are taken by professional photographers with all the benefits of expensive lighting, makeup, and clothing.

Screen Time vs. Social Media Use

In 2019, researchers at the University of Oxford made headlines when they failed to find any meaningful connection between screen time and poor mental health. In 2022, researchers at San Diego State University led by Jean M. Twenge analyzed the same data. They discussed their findings in an editorial:

> The paper's definition of "screen time" included watching TV or simply owning a computer as well as healthy social interaction such as talking with friends on the phone. . . . Does the story change when we limit the analysis to social media, which is where teenagers gather most often?
>
> It does, enormously. In a new paper, we used the same advanced statistical technique and found that the link between social media use and poor mental health for girls was 10 times as large as what the Oxford paper identified for "screen time."
>
> The new study shows that, for girls in particular, the correlation between mental health and social media use is larger than that between mental health and binge drinking, early sexual activity, hard drug use, being suspended from school, marijuana use, lack of exercise, being stopped by police, and carrying a weapon.

Jean Twenge, Jonathan Haidt, and Kevin Cummins, "Opinion: Social Media Is Riskier for Kids than 'Screen Time,'" *Washington Post*, February 16, 2022. www.washingtonpost.com.

Although more teen girls than teen boys say Instagram makes them feel worse about themselves, Facebook's research shows that boys are also negatively affected by the comparisons they make on the photo-sharing app. The Facebook study found that 40 percent of teen boys experience negative social comparison when using Instagram. These negative comparisons resulted in 14 percent of teen boys reporting feeling worse about themselves after using the app, with 2 percent saying they felt a great deal worse. Some also maintained that if they did not create flawless posts, they would face instant criticism. "I just feel on the edge a lot of the time," one teen boy told the researchers. "It's like you can be called out for anything you do. One wrong move. One wrong step."[31]

More Evidence of Harm

Facebook's internal research shocked the public, but it did not come as a surprise to other researchers in the field. "Facebook's own research confirms what many academic researchers had been saying for years—that for some people, especially teen girls, social media can harm mental health, and that the rise in depression and self-harm among teens since 2010 might be caused by the increasing popularity of social media,"[32] writes Jean M. Twenge, a psychology professor at San Diego State University.

Twenge and her colleagues have published several papers documenting the impact of social media on teens. In a 2018 study of screen time among teens, Twenge's team found that after one hour of use per day, "more hours of daily screen time were associated with lower psychological well-being, including less curiosity, lower self-control, more distractibility, more difficulty making friends, less emotional stability, being more difficult to care for, and inability to finish tasks."[33] The more hours teens spent on their devices, the higher the incidence of mental health problems. Compared to teens who used their devices one hour or less per day, those who averaged more than seven hours of screen time were twice as likely to have ever been diagnosed with depression or anxiety, treated by a

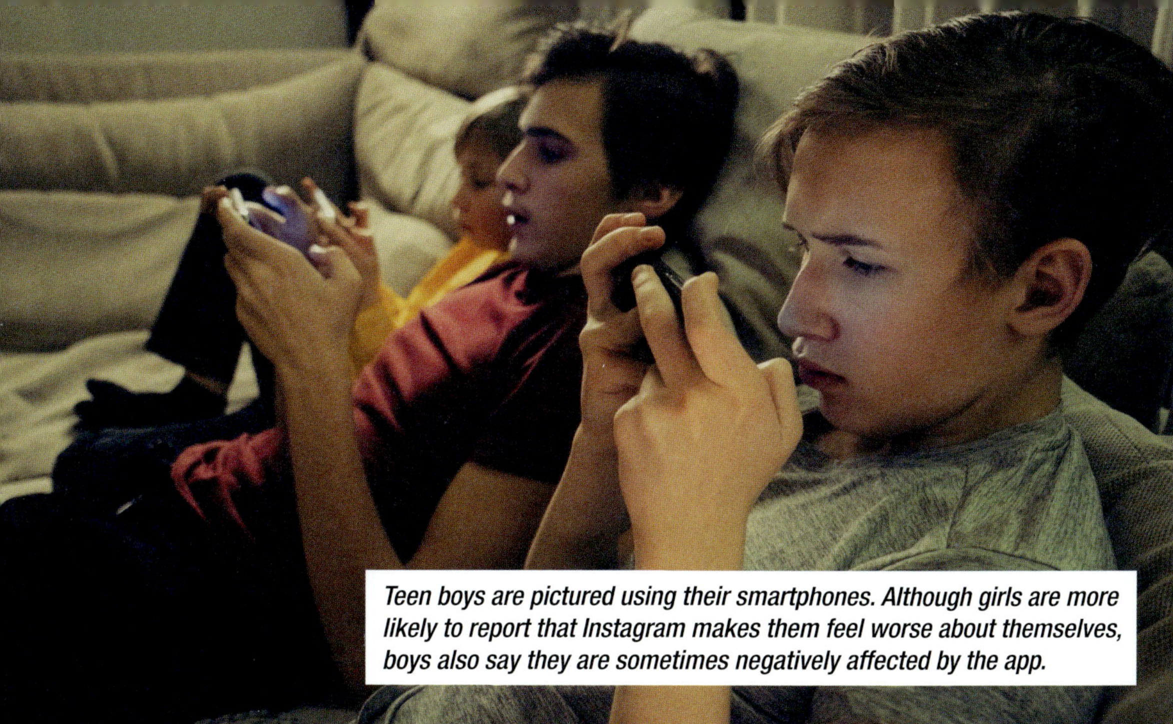

Teen boys are pictured using their smartphones. Although girls are more likely to report that Instagram makes them feel worse about themselves, boys also say they are sometimes negatively affected by the app.

mental health professional, or taken medication for a psychological or behavioral issue in the previous twelve months.

A 2022 study by Twenge and her colleagues found that teen girls are at risk from all social media, not just Instagram. The researchers analyzed data from more than 350,000 adolescents from three surveys: the Youth Risk Behavior Surveillance System, a biennial survey administered by the Centers for Disease Control and Prevention to a nationally representative sample of US students in ninth to twelfth grade; the Monitoring the Future project, which, since 1991, has annually surveyed a nationally representative sample of US students in eighth and tenth grade; and the Millennium Cohort Study, a nationally representative sample of UK adolescents born in 2000 and 2001. The researchers found a consistent and substantial association between poor mental health and social media use among teen girls. "These associations were stronger than links between mental health and binge drinking, sexual assault, obesity, and hard drug use," write the researchers. "These associations may have substantial practical significance as many countries are experiencing rising rates of depression, anxiety, and suicide among teenagers and young adults."[34]

CHAPTER THREE

The Lure of Online Gaming

Jack, a sixteen-year-old student from Grand Rapids, Michigan, was eight years old when he got his first video game console, a Nintendo DS. Gaming soon became his favorite pastime. "Up until I was in the 6th grade, I'd play games on my Nintendo DS for hours every day," he says. "Not much changed after that, but the DS got replaced by the Wii U. I loved gaming because I could just switch off while playing. It didn't take much brainpower and it would keep me entertained for hours."[35]

Although he played a lot, Jack was able to control his participation in offline gaming. Once he started playing online games, however, things began to change. "Things got worse when I bought an Xbox One," he says. The problem with online gaming is that it contributes to FOMO. Online gamers often play competitively with other people. Because they are involved with others, either competing against them or playing on the same team, online gamers often find it hard to quit playing on their own schedule. Their loyalty to the team and the sense of belonging can keep them playing even when they know they should stop. If they leave, they feel they are missing out on something important. This is what happened to Jack. "It became impossible to disconnect from my devices,"[36] he recalls.

A Day in the Life of a Gaming Addict

Jack recognized that gaming was taking over his life. "I realized gaming was a problem because I started spending more time in front of a screen instead of doing what I really loved—

playing the guitar. I began spending more time at home playing games than going out with friends," he says. He described his typical day when he was gaming: "I would wake up and play video games for a couple of hours while still in bed. I'd get breakfast and come back up to my room to play more games. After lunch, I'd get back to gaming in my room or on my DS. Then I'd spend time playing games on my phone. Finally, I'd head back to bed." The long hours spent gaming took a toll on Jack. "I started sleeping less and found myself not enjoying life as much. I became depressed and anxious,"[37] he remembers.

A Widespread Problem

Jack was far from alone in his struggles with video game addiction. According to a 2021 study by the Entertainment Software Association, the trade association of the US video game industry, 227 million Americans play video games, including 75 percent of youths under eighteen. The WHO estimates that 3 to 4 percent of gamers are addicted to the activity. That means between 6.8 million and 9 million video game players are addicted in the United States, including up to 1.8 million players under the age of eighteen.

Some experts believe the WHO estimate is too high. A study by researchers at Oxford University in England, led by Andrew K. Przybylski, found that no more than 1 percent of the 18,932 gamers surveyed met all the criteria for internet gaming disorder (IGD). Nevertheless, the study suggests that with the current number of gamers in the United States, 2.27 million—including 454,000 under the age of eighteen—could be addicted. "This represents a large cohort of people struggling with what could be clinically dysregulated [uncontrolled] behavior,"[38] state the researchers.

Defining Gaming Addiction

Przybylski and his team used a definition of *gaming addiction* proposed by the American Psychiatric Association (APA). The definition states that video game players may have IGD if they exhibit five or more of the following criteria within a twelve-month period:

1. Preoccupation with Internet games. (The individual thinks about previous gaming activity or anticipates playing the next game; Internet gaming becomes the dominant activity in daily life.)

2. Withdrawal symptoms when Internet gaming is taken away. (These symptoms are typically described as irritability, anxiety, or sadness, but there are no physical signs of pharmacological withdrawal.)

3. Tolerance—the need to spend increasing amounts of time engaged in Internet games.

4. Unsuccessful attempts to control the participation in Internet games.

5. Continued excessive use of Internet games despite knowledge of psychosocial problems.

6. Has deceived family members, therapists, or others regarding the amount of Internet gaming.

7. Use of Internet games to escape or relieve a negative mood (e.g., feelings of helplessness, guilt, anxiety).

8. Loss of interest in previous hobbies and entertainment as a result of, and with the exception of, Internet games.

9. Has jeopardized or lost a significant relationship, job, or educational or career opportunity because of participation in Internet games.[39]

The definition of IGD is broader than its name suggests, according to Professor Gentile of Iowa State University. "Despite its

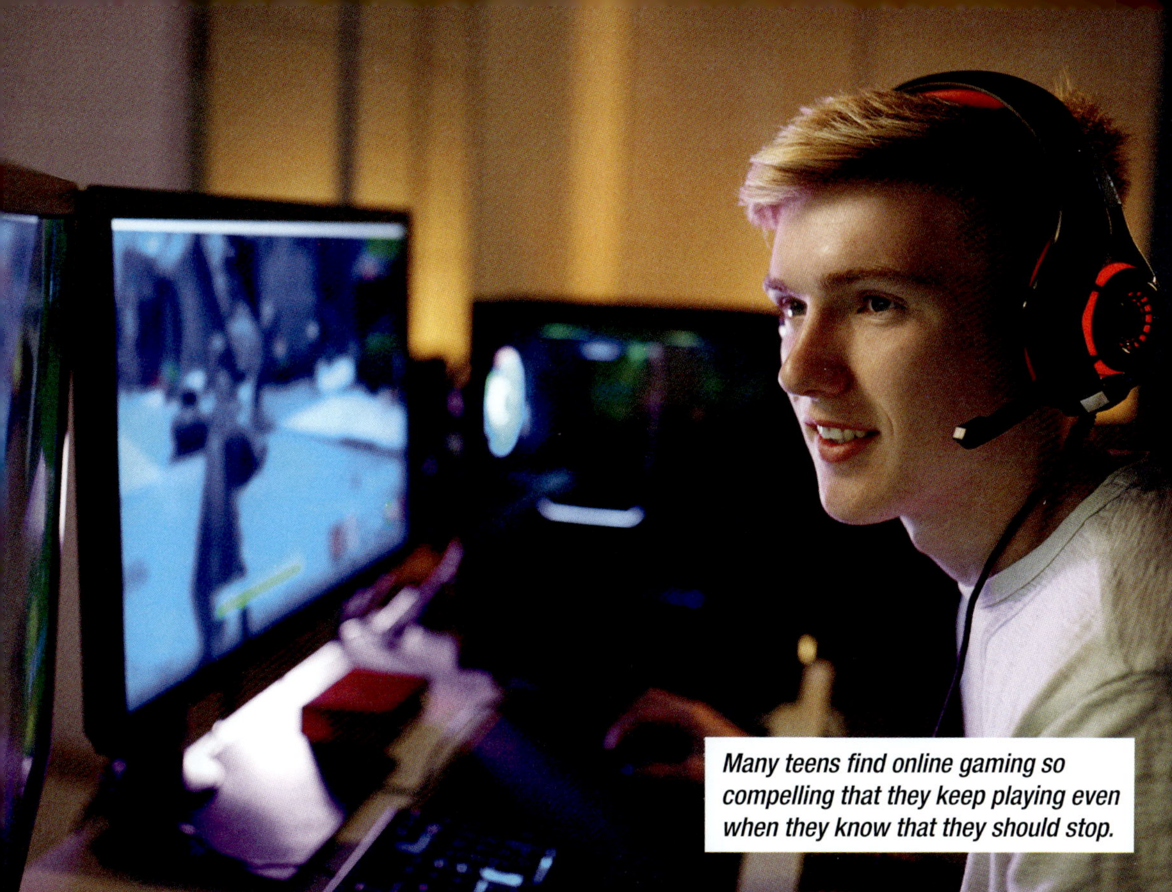

name, IGD does not require that individuals exhibit symptoms of addiction solely with online video games," Gentile says. "Problematic use can occur in both offline and online settings."[40]

Przybylski's team found that 2.4 percent of the study participants reported having experienced five or more of the symptoms on the APA list, suggesting that they met the criteria for IGD. The researchers acknowledged that this 2.4 percent was "a level close to the 3.1% estimated in a comprehensive recent meta-analysis"[41] conducted by researchers at Texas A&M University. The 2.4 percent figure would suggest that 5.4 million Americans, including 1 million gamers under the age of eighteen, meet the criteria for IGD.

To arrive at their final 1 percent tally, Przybylski's team only counted those participants who met five or more of the APA criteria and "reported that they suffered significant distress due to gaming." This last qualifier, they explained, was added to

A Gamer Struggles with Suicidal Thoughts

Anthony got his first gaming console at age seven. "I absolutely fell in love with it," he recalls. Later, however, his gaming began to destroy his life. He explains:

> During school I was bullied a lot for being gay, so video games became my escape. I could be accepted and validated in a virtual world, while the real world felt harsh and unsafe for a gay kid raised in the nineties. Doing well at first person shooters made me feel in control and gave me a purpose.
>
> As I became a teenager, I started to isolate myself more and more from my peers and family. Video games became the only thing I enjoyed doing. . . .
>
> I was lonely and depressed. I was exhausted of having no goals or vision for my life. I felt I had been wasting my life in a virtual world, while the real world was out there waiting for me. When I started to experience suicidal feelings, I knew I needed help.
>
> I began seeing a therapist and she encouraged me to unplug from video games. . . . So I took a leap of faith. I sold and donated ALL of my gaming equipment.

Anthony, "Suicidal Gamer Escapes to a Life Worth Living," Game Quitters, May 21, 2020. https://gamequitters.com.

distinguish between those players who have a healthy love of gaming from those who have an unhealthy dependence on it:

> This guidance acknowledges that dysregulated [uncontrolled] gaming is characterized by significant distress, a nuance that may discriminate passion from pathology. Many players may experience a feature of Internet gaming disorder, for example, a preoccupation with a new game that distracts from other responsibilities. Much in the same way a sports fan might feel distracted at work if his or her team reaches the finals, feeling this way may be typical

among those for whom gaming is a favored hobby. Such experiences are not necessarily pathological if unaccompanied by significant distress.[42]

A Case of IGD

The symptoms of IGD—including significant distress—were all present in the life of Tom, a man who posted his story on Game Quitters, a website that supports gamers who are addicted to gaming. When Tom was six years old, his family gave him and his older brother an Xbox. "From then on, . . . gaming was my main source of entertainment," says Tom, now twenty-three, describing the onset of his first symptoms—preoccupation with internet games and a loss of interest in previous hobbies and entertainment as a result of gaming. "It was how I de-stressed; it was how I passed time; it was how I interacted with my two brothers and the few friends I made. I didn't play outside much. I never learned how to ride a bike or swim. And my visits to the beach decreased significantly."[43]

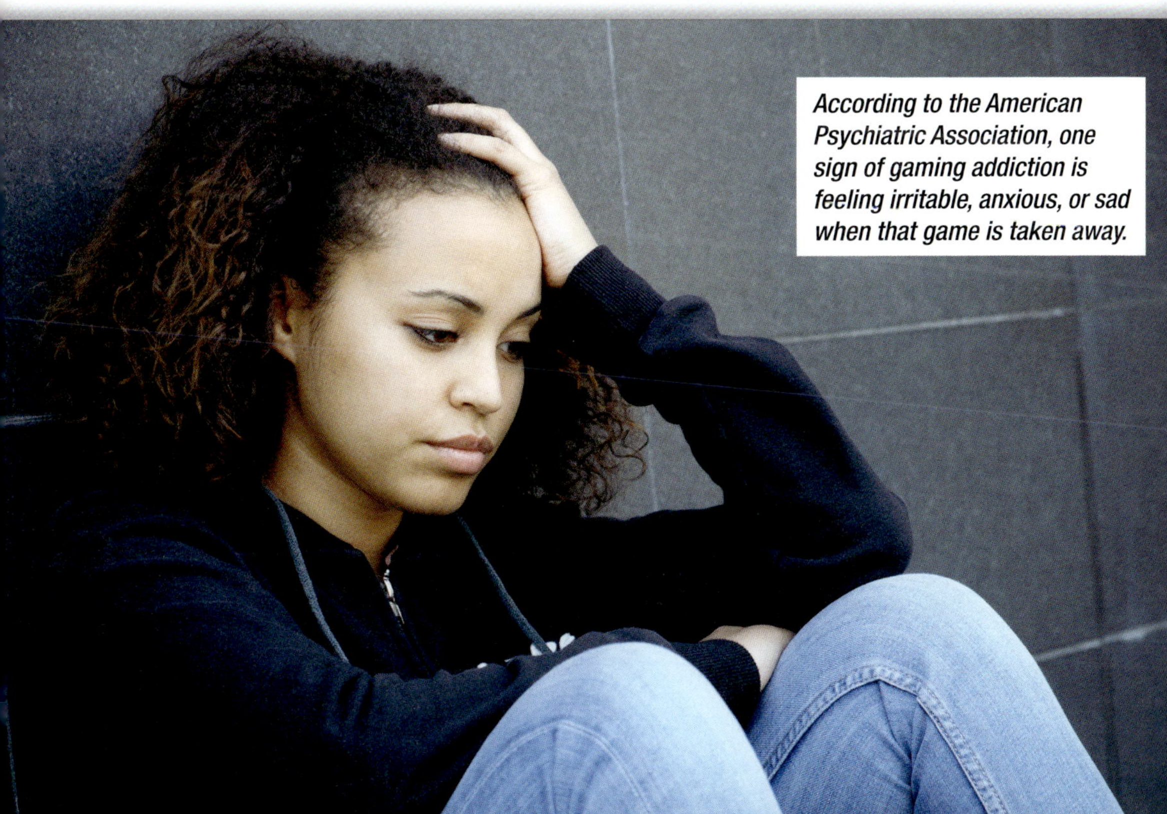

According to the American Psychiatric Association, one sign of gaming addiction is feeling irritable, anxious, or sad when that game is taken away.

Tom felt more comfortable in the virtual world than in the real one. While still in elementary school, gaming began to affect his personal relationships—another criterion of IGD. "I have a very distinct memory of some time in elementary school when two girls in the neighborhood came to my house to invite me out to play, and I pretended to be sick so I could avoid interacting," Tom recalls. "Instead, I played video games."[44]

In middle school, Tom realized that he had to hide his addiction to video games if he were going to have any friends at all. "To impress people and relate to them, I ended up developing a lying problem," he says. "I would tell people grand stories of what I did in my free time and how active a person I was, when in reality, when I got off the bus from school, I went to my room and played Halo, Runescape, Mass Effect, Command and Conquer, etc. I told people I hunted (I'd never held a gun in my life). I told people I played lacrosse (never held a lacrosse stick in my life)."[45] Misleading others about the extent of his gaming was another sign of Tom's developing IGD.

In high school, Tom made friends with other gamers and began to adopt their habits, playing longer hours and experimenting with other games. Even though he was not particularly good at math, he began to take science, technology, engineering, and mathematics courses just to be around people who accepted him. When he finished high school, he decided to study electrical engineering in college. Making life decisions based on a habit or behavior is also a sign of a growing dependency. "Needless to say, all the math courses and engineering courses were really difficult for me, and I struggled through my freshman year," Tom says. "All the way, I de-stressed with video games."[46] Using video games to escape or relieve a negative mood is another sign of addiction.

The WHO Recognizes Video Game Addiction

The WHO's *International Classification of Diseases,* 11th revision, officially recognizes compulsive video game playing as a behavioral addiction. The manual provides health care professionals with a definition of the condition, which it calls *gaming disorder*:

> Gaming disorder is characterized by a pattern of persistent or recurrent gaming behavior ("digital gaming" or "video-gaming"), which may be online (i.e., over the Internet) or offline, manifested by:
>
> 1. impaired control over gaming (e.g., onset, frequency, intensity, duration, termination, context);
>
> 2. increasing priority given to gaming to the extent that gaming takes precedence over other life interests and daily activities; and
>
> 3. continuation or escalation of gaming despite the occurrence of negative consequences. The behavior pattern is of sufficient severity to result in significant impairment in personal, family, social, educational, occupational or other important areas of functioning.
>
> The pattern of gaming behavior may be continuous or episodic and recurrent. The gaming behavior and other features are normally evident over a period of at least 12 months in order for a diagnosis to be assigned, although the required duration may be shortened if all diagnostic requirements are met and symptoms are severe.

World Health Organization, "6C51 Gaming Disorder," ICD-11 for Mortality and Morbidity Statistics, April 2019. https://icd.who.int.

Realizing that gaming was interfering with his schoolwork, Tom decided to make a change in his life. "My sophomore year, I ended up leaving school to try to explore new things, but I mostly spent my time at home playing video games."[47] This stage of Tom's life revealed another symptom: continued excessive use of gaming despite knowledge of psychosocial problems.

Finally, Tom decided to give up gaming. "I decided to experiment with quitting video games, having identified them as a key point of failure in my freshman year," he says. He tried deleting his Steam account, selling his gaming laptop, and even took a more drastic step. "One night, I realized how far I'd fallen back into my addiction, and I had what I can only describe as a panic attack," he remembers. "I was so afraid that video games would be all I ever did with my life that I intentionally water damaged our Xbox 360 to stop myself from playing it."[48] But no matter what he did, he always returned to gaming. This behavior exposed one of the clearest symptoms of addiction: loss of control, or relapse.

In 2020, Tom decided to seek help to end his addiction. "I started seeing a therapist for the depression and anxiety that I believe are heavily rooted in my background in gaming." Even under the care of a professional, Tom experienced relapses. However, he began to explore other interests. "I'm going to start posting on Medium, covering the subjects of video game addiction, Internet addiction, and switching career paths after college," he says. "I feel like a creative person with a lot of drive and motivation and energy who has just been held hostage by video games all their life. I have a lot of regret for wasting my entire childhood, but I'm glad that, at 23, I'm able to move on in a healthier direction."[49]

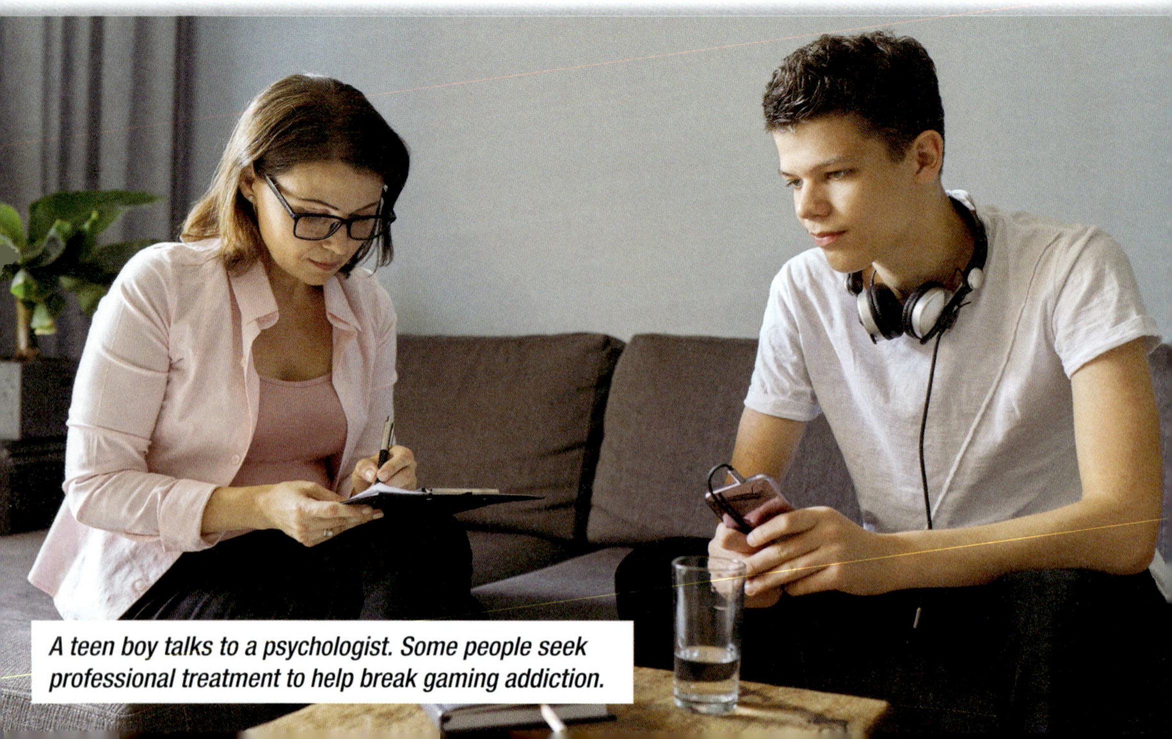

A teen boy talks to a psychologist. Some people seek professional treatment to help break gaming addiction.

Recognition of Gaming Disorder

The APA has included IGD in the research appendix of its *Diagnostic and Statistical Manual of Mental Disorders,* fifth edition. The organization is holding off fully recognizing IGD as a disorder, pending more clinical research and experience. In the meantime, however, the WHO has included gaming disorder (GD) in the eleventh revision of its *International Classification of Diseases.* The WHO also gave the disorder its own diagnosis code.

This recognition of GD is important for several reasons. It gives medical professionals a standard for diagnosing video game addiction. It means that researchers can study the phenomenon more efficiently because they can all be working with a single definition of the disorder, regardless of what country they are in. It could also encourage health insurance companies to pay for treatment, which would increase access for those needing help. As Gentile explains,

> There are about 40 million children in the U.S. If . . . 8 percent of them would classify as having gaming disorder, that's over 3 million children in the U.S. today causing serious damage to their lives because of the way they're playing. . . . That's a lot of kids who would benefit from getting help but up until now haven't been able to because it hasn't been considered a real diagnosis.[50]

More than 225 million Americans play video games on consoles, computers, tablets, and phones. According to the Entertainment Software Association, 90 percent of gamers say their hobby brings them joy through play, and 87 percent say it provides stress relief. However, a small percentage of gamers—between 1 percent and 8 percent—cannot control their game play and experience significant distress as a result. Their pastime has become a compulsion, and it is harming them. They are addicted. Addiction to video games is one of the major components of screen addiction.

CHAPTER FOUR

Designed to Engage

Whether engaged with social media, video games, texting, or streaming content, people who are addicted to screens tend to blame themselves for being too weak to control their activities. Many do not realize that their choices are being influenced by features built into the software they are using. These features are designed to keep users interacting with the apps, drawing them toward addiction.

The makers of free apps such as Instagram, Facebook, YouTube, Candy Crush Saga, and thousands of others all earn money from advertisers. These advertisers pay the companies for the right to place advertisements within the app's content. Each company normally is paid on the basis of how many users view an ad, so it is to the company's benefit to keep users engaged with the app for as long as possible. The longer users are engaged, the more ads they will see, and the more money the content provider will earn. "In order to get the next round of funding, in order to get your stock price up, the amount of time that people spend on your app has to go up," explains Aza Raskin, a software engineer who formerly worked at Mozilla, the company behind the Firefox web browser. "So, when you put that much pressure on that one number, you're going to start trying to invent new ways of getting people to stay hooked."[51]

Raskin himself played a pivotal role in the development of one of the most habit-forming features of mobile apps: the ability for the user to view a never-ending stream of content by simply swiping across the face of a device. This feature is known as infinite scroll. Because scrolling requires minimal effort, users can lose track of how much time is passing as they watch the content streaming across their screens. "If you don't give your brain time to catch up with your impulses, you just keep scrolling,"[52] explains Raskin. According to Andrew Keller, a vice president overseeing user experience at Facebook, the average person scrolls through about 300 feet (91 m)—the length of a football field—of photos, memes, videos, tweets, and posts every day.

One such user is Rebecca Fishbein, an author in Brooklyn, New York. "The first thing I do when I wake up is check Twitter on my phone. I know this is a bad habit, . . . because my day starts off with an endless scroll," says Fishbein. "The mindless scroll isn't limited to my mornings. I scroll through my Instagram feed at parties. I click through Tinder in line at the grocery store."[53]

Fishbein is not alone in her response to the feature, nor is her behavior an unfortunate accident. The feature was designed to overpower the ability of users to place limits on how much time they spend on their devices, keeping them on the app for as long as possible. "The scrolling doesn't draw us in, but it keeps us there for much longer than we might be if the feeds ended, or if we had to click buttons to reveal new content," says Adam Alter, a professor at New York University. "People tend to function on autopilot until something inside their heads or in the world around them subtly or explicitly suggests it's time to move on. Reaching the end of a feed is one such cue; removing the end point short-circuits that cue."[54]

Infinite scroll is not the only feature designed to keep users engaged with their devices. "Behind every screen on your phone, there are generally like literally a thousand (user experience) engineers that have worked on this thing to try to make it maximally addicting," says Raskin. "It's as if they're taking behavioral cocaine and just sprinkling it all over your interface, and that's the thing that keeps you like coming back and back and back."[55]

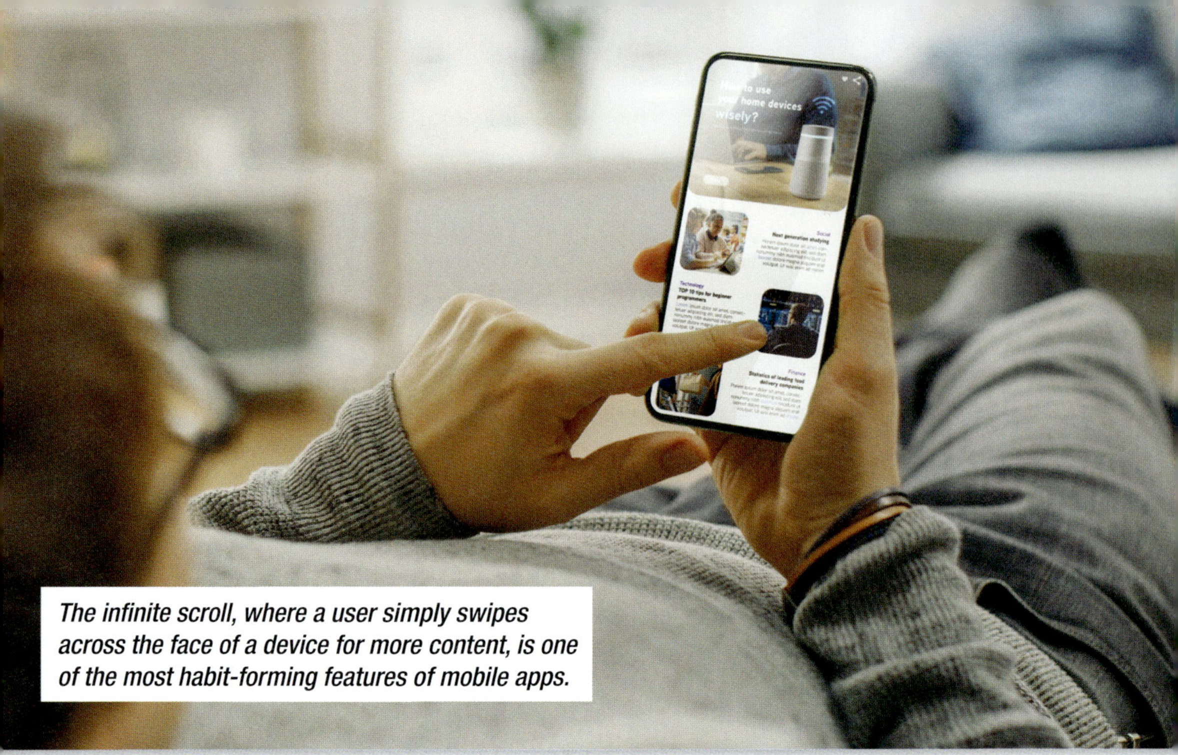

The infinite scroll, where a user simply swipes across the face of a device for more content, is one of the most habit-forming features of mobile apps.

Another feature that acts as a magnet for screen overuse is the ability to approve of posted material using icons such as a thumbs-up signs, hearts, or emojis. Many users become obsessed with how much attention their social media posts are receiving because they see their "likes" and "loves" as signs of their own self-worth. Leah Pearlman, who helped develop the "like" button when she worked at Facebook, ironically fell prey to to the feature. "When I need validation—I go to check Facebook," she says. "I'm feeling lonely, 'Let me check my phone.' I'm feeling insecure, 'Let me check my phone.'" She found that she was constantly checking her devices throughout the day. "Suddenly," she recalls, "I thought I'm actually also kind of addicted to the feedback."[56]

Affecting the Brain's Chemistry

Like infinite scroll, social media feedback bypasses the reasoning part of the brain, stimulating a more primitive area of the organ. This region releases a substance known as dopamine, which is a chemical the nervous system uses to send messages between nerve cells. Dopamine creates feelings of pleasure and well-being deep within the brain. Normally, the brain releases dopamine to reward behaviors that help ensure a person's survival, such as eating, drinking, or socializing. As such, dopamine is part of what is known as the body's reward circuit. The brain can also release dopamine to reward a success or achievement, from figuring out a word in a crossword puzzle to making a winning shot in a basketball game.

Scientists have found that the brain even releases dopamine when a person receives positive feedback on a social media post or even comes across a pleasing picture while scrolling through social media. Former Facebook engineer Justin Rosenstein calls the dopamine spikes caused by social media "bright dings of pseudo-pleasure"[57] because the rewards are not given for real achievements, only for social media feedback. Regardless of the reason, the chemical response is real and powerful. "The same brain pathways get stimulated as they do in a chemical addiction," says psychologist Joshua Ehrlich. "It really is an addiction, and we're wired for this."[58]

Researchers have observed that social media's effect on brain chemistry is similar to that of gambling—another activity that can become addictive. When gamblers play blackjack, roulette, or slot machines, they usually both win and lose. The losses usually exceed the wins, but the wins cause a release of dopamine that gives the gambler a feeling of pleasure or well-being. These spikes in dopamine can keep a gambler playing for long periods.

Psychologists call the occasional wins that occur in gambling and other activities "intermittent variable rewards." The uncertainty regarding if or when a reward will be received is essential to the release of dopamine. The brain only releases dopamine when a success or achievement follows a period of uncertainty. If an activity always results in a success, there would be no need to reward the body for succeeding.

Facing Social Media Addictions

Author Dana Bowman discovered that she was addicted to what she calls "mindless scrolling." She told her story to *Psychology Today*:

> Every night I found myself scrolling through endless videos. . . . I loved it. All those tiny videos, just quick little nips of sparkle or pathos or food porn; it latched onto me and I just kept scrolling. And scrolling.
>
> And scrolling. . . .
>
> Social media is the fast food of screens for the eyes. But, no matter how much we are aware of this, we can get sucked into the scrolling. Why?
>
> For one, social media changes the brain. It can trigger a dopamine hit, which ultimately is unable to be filled. It can engender chronic distraction, wreaking havoc on our peace, our self-control, our priorities. It can take that initial positive attribute of connection and communication, and break it down into isolation and perfectionism in relationships. And, it really feeds my inner addict.
>
> I no longer regarded social media as a tool to help me achieve something: better communication, information, learning, a better headspace. Instead, the device in itself was the end game. It was a numbing blind alley. It didn't expedite. It ended.

Dana Bowman, "My Name Is Dana, and I'm Addicted to Mindless Scrolling," *Highly Functioning Is Highly Dangerous* (blog), *Psychology Today*, September 6, 2020. www.psychologytoday.com.

Like gambling, social media offers intermittent variable rewards in the form of "likes," "loves," "shares," and "retweets." Social media users anticipate such feedback, but they never know when the reactions might come. As a result, they keep checking their devices. "Social media sites are chock-a-block [stuffed full] with unpredictable rewards," says Professor Griffiths of Nottingham Trent University's International Gaming Research Unit. "They are trying to grab users' attentions . . . to make social media users create a routine and habitually check their screens."[59]

The dopamine rewards that users receive from their social media activity causes them to engage further, posting more content in the hope of receiving more rewards. "Social reward, in the form of likes and comments, is very reinforcing," says Erin A. Vogel, a social psychologist. "We feel good when we get social reward, so we keep posting."[60] The process of posting, receiving rewards, and posting again creates an endless loop that can be addicting.

Failure to receive positive reactions to a social media post can also feed screen addiction. If a post does not result in the hoped-for response, the user can experience anxiety. "Consciously and unconsciously, most people feed off of the energy created by a high level of likes; this can feel fabulous when the number of likes is high, yet a low number of likes can lead to feelings of sadness and negativity," says Carla Marie Manly, a clinical psychologist. To overcome these negative feelings, users often do not take a break from their devices. Instead, they try to post something new that will prove popular. "The resulting highs and lows can lead to an addictive pattern of making posts geared toward getting likes in order to feel the invigorating rush,"[61] Manly says.

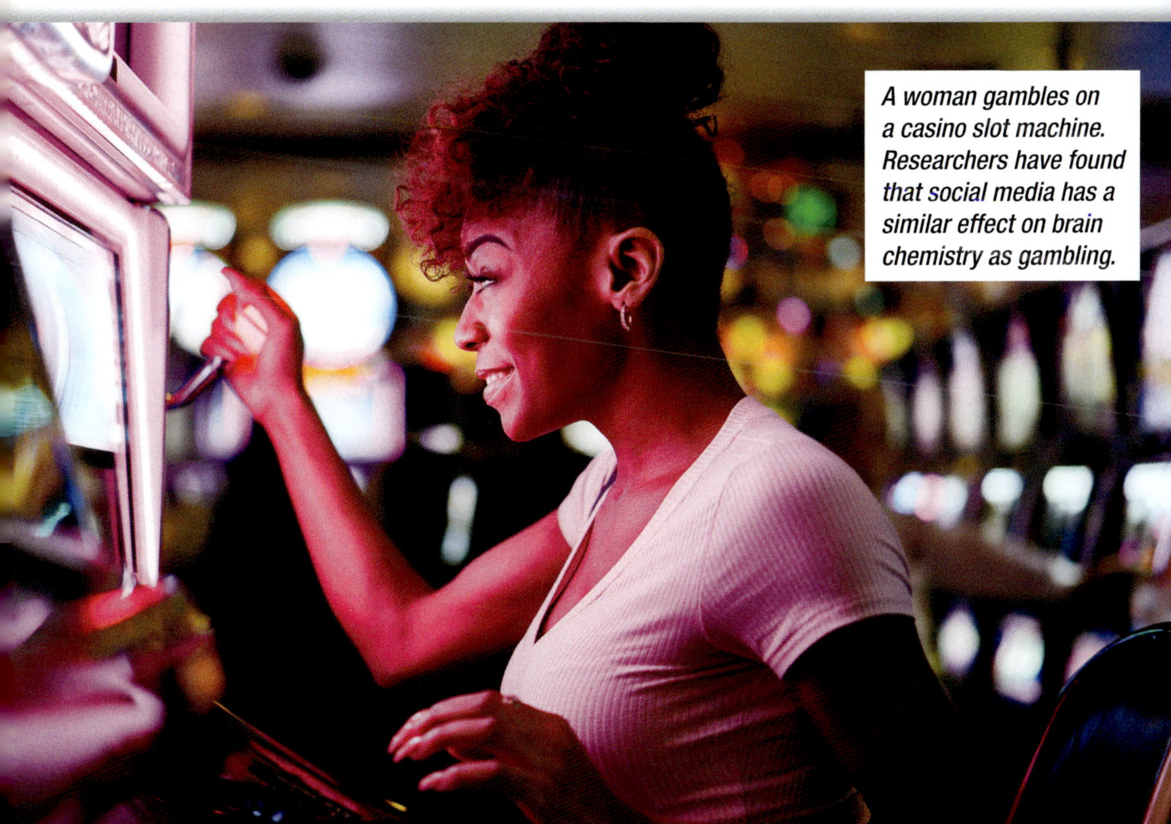

A woman gambles on a casino slot machine. Researchers have found that social media has a similar effect on brain chemistry as gambling.

The Lure of Loot Boxes

Intermittent variable rewards also play a role in making video games addictive. Not only does successful game play flood the brain with dopamine, as with success at other sports and games, but a feature known as a loot box employs the concept of intermittent variable rewards to entice players into spending additional money on their games. Available in games such as *Fortnite, Overwatch*, and *League of Legends*, loot boxes contain virtual items called loot that enhance game play, allowing players to customize their avatars or automatically advance in a video game. Costing anywhere from $1 to $300, the items in loot boxes typically cannot be earned with game play; they must be purchased separately.

The addictive feature of loot boxes is that players do not know what is in the box before they pay to open it. Like a slot machine or roulette wheel, loot boxes use intermittent variable rewards to hook players into buying them. In a 2021 report by the University of Plymouth and the University of Wolverhampton in the United Kingdom, researchers concluded that loot boxes "are structurally and psychologically akin to gambling."[62] Their survey of 13,115 active gamers found that just 5 percent of gamers generate half the entire revenue from loot boxes. "We have demonstrated that at-risk individuals, such as problem gamblers, gamers, and young people, make disproportionate contributions to loot box revenues,"[63] says James Close, one of the report's authors.

Video game makers and social media companies both know that features of their software can stimulate the production of dopamine and lure users into becoming addict-

Hooked on Loot Boxes

Studies show that buying loot boxes stimulates the brain in the same way that gambling does, and this stimulation can prove addicting. One gamer who got hooked on loot boxes goes by the handle CadenceLikesVGs. Her favorite game is *Path of Exile*, an online role-playing game that releases new loot boxes every three months. The loot boxes enable the players to customize their character's gear, which is an important element for serious players. Although each loot box costs only about $3, a player may have to open many boxes before getting the desired loot. CadenceLikesVGs says she has spent up to $400 to obtain a highly desired item. She describes her addiction:

> When your brain works like mine, you can't stop. There is always the little voice of the back of your head that goes, "Yeah, no, man, you should've quit like 30 boxes ago," but even when you're telling yourself to stop, you're still clicking buy, and you're still opening boxes. . . .
>
> People tend to jump on the loot boxes thinking they'll get a deal, but that's not how gambling works. The house always wins.

Quoted in Makena Kelly, "How Loot Boxes Hooked Gamers and Left Regulators Spinning," The Verge, February19, 2019. www.theverge.com.

ed to their products. The situation recalls the way that cigarette makers during the mid-twentieth century knew that cigarettes were addictive but withheld that information from the public to keep selling their products. At the time, 54 percent of Americans were smokers. Only after the US surgeon general issued warnings about tobacco products and Congress banned their advertising on television did the public begin to turn away from smoking, with the number dwindling to just 13 percent in 2018. Some lawmakers believe it is time to take similar action against the addictive features of electronic devices, perhaps outlawing infinite scrolling, likes and other feedback, and loot boxes. Otherwise, the number of people struggling with screen addiction is likely to grow.

CHAPTER FIVE

Overcoming Screen Addiction

The first and often the hardest step to overcoming any addiction is for users to admit they have a problem. This is particularly hard when it comes to a behavioral addiction because addicted individuals see so many other people doing the same thing they are doing—whether it is shopping, gambling, eating, or any other behavior known to be addictive—without any ill effects. It is even more difficult with screen addiction because many people remain skeptical that it is an addiction at all. Yet many mental health professionals, and even the WHO, recognize that it is. Although billions of people can use their devices for several hours a day without ill effects, a certain percentage cannot. They lose control over their behavior. They are addicted.

Once these users recognize they have lost control of their screen usage, they must take concrete steps to change their lives and break free of the habit. For people addicted to drugs or alcohol, the most effective solution is to give up all mood-altering substances completely. This is because even a small amount of an intoxicating substance can trigger a relapse into addiction. But this solution—total abstinence—is not practical for many behavioral addictions. A person with gambling addiction can give up gambling completely because it is not essential to life. But a person with an eating disorder cannot give up eating, and a person with a shopping addiction would find it almost impossible to stop purchasing items. For this reason, treatment of behavioral addictions often focuses on modifying rather than eliminating the behavior.

Modification is the most practical approach for screen addiction. Although people whose livelihoods do not involve working with digital devices might be able to end their contact with screens completely, for most people, total abstinence from electronics is not practical. They need to be able to use computers and even cell phones to survive in the digital economy. "To quit cold turkey would impose an enormous cost on virtually anyone who needs to manage a bank account, communicate with loved ones, call for a ride, work remotely, or perform countless other everyday tasks," says Arthur C. Brooks, a professor of management practice at the Harvard Business School. "So the proper approach is to find the right level to which we should aspire."[64]

Do-It-Yourself Treatment

Many people with screen addiction attempt to modify their behavior themselves. One popular technique they use is called mindfulness, a Buddhist concept based on concentrating fully on the present moment. "The best way to counteract mindless scrolling is with mindful scrolling," says Brooks. "Set times each day or week to look at your smartphone and really focus on it. Don't do anything else; be all about the phone for those minutes, as if it were your job." Concentrating on their devices for a brief period allows the user to drastically reduce screen time while still having time to respond to important messages and posts. "Besides making addiction easier to beat, . . . such a practice might also show you how little you actually enjoy staring at your phone,"[65] explains Brooks.

Some do-it-yourselfers find it hard to enforce the limits they place on their screen time, so they turn to the devices themselves for help. They download apps that monitor and limit the amount of time they spend on particular websites, such as

Instagram, TikTok, or Facebook. These timer apps allow users to gradually reduce their screen time, from hours a day, to an hour, and finally to minutes. Like mindfulness, setting limits on screen time allows users to remain in touch with friends and family while eliminating overuse.

Time-limiting apps often keep a log of online activity. Seeing the time spent on various apps and websites often strengthens a user's resolve to cut back on screen time. Detailed records of online use can also make users more accountable for their behavior. The apps do not accept excuses, and users must take full responsibility for their actions. If they have trouble sticking to their limits, users can share the time logs with friends or family members who can support them in their attempts to break their addiction.

Deleting the Apps

Gradually reducing screen time, even with the help of timer apps, does not work for everyone. Jack, a teen who struggled with gaming addiction, is one such person. "For me, there's no such thing as moderation," he says. "I had to sell my DS and all of the games for my consoles. I even got rid of all the games on my computer."[66]

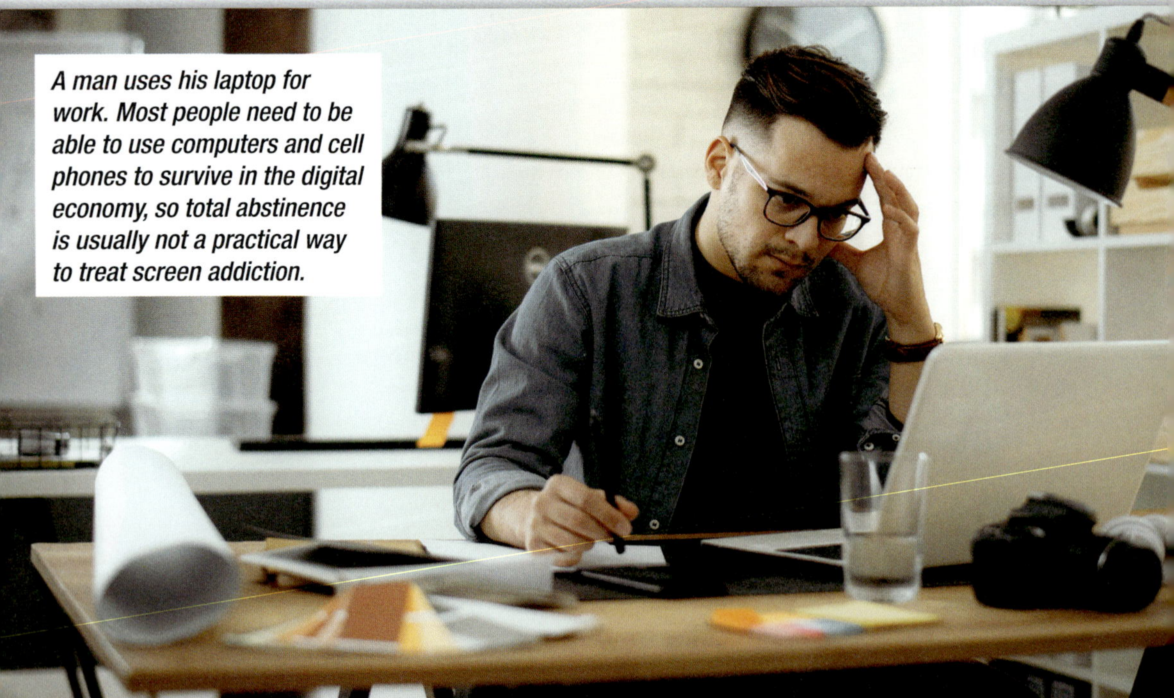

A man uses his laptop for work. Most people need to be able to use computers and cell phones to survive in the digital economy, so total abstinence is usually not a practical way to treat screen addiction.

Deleting apps can be an abrupt change, creating a void in the user's life. Adapting to the change can be difficult, unless the user fills the void with offline activities. Jack filled some of the time he recovered by playing the guitar. "I sold my Xbox One and finally bought that second guitar I wanted," he recalls. He offers friendly advice to others who are struggling with the same problem. "What really helped me was replacing urges [to play video games] with going outside or hanging out with a friend," he says. "It's a lot easier to overcome the cravings if you get yourself out of the house."[67]

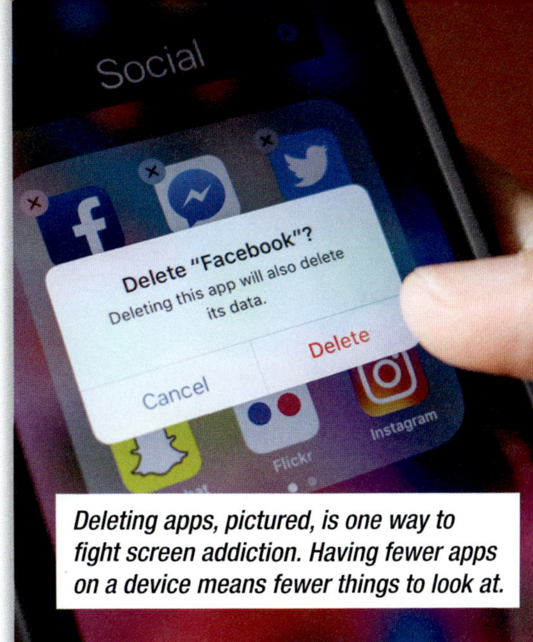

Deleting apps, pictured, is one way to fight screen addiction. Having fewer apps on a device means fewer things to look at.

Deleting an app does not mean a person cannot go back to it, of course. The user can simply reinstall the app. To make this more difficult, some people install apps that block access to certain websites. These apps can also be uninstalled, but they are designed to slow down users and make sure they really want access to the sites they blocked. Sometimes this extra layer of accountability is enough to prevent a relapse.

Seeking Professional Help

In many cases, a screen addiction is so strong that do-it-yourself techniques do not solve the problem. In such cases, the addicted person might need to see a mental health professional for counseling, either in person or in online sessions. Because screen addiction is not yet recognized by the APA, treatment might not be covered by health insurance. Instead, the user will have to pay out of pocket, with costs typically being between $100 and $200 for a weekly fifty-minute session.

A common treatment for behavioral addictions such as screen addiction is known as cognitive behavioral therapy (CBT). In this

Four Steps to Stop Using Social Media

In this excerpt, Matt Glowiak, a licensed clinical professional counselor, offers four steps to stop using social media:

1. Be Strict About Limiting Your Time
   First and foremost, you should restrict your time on social media. In the very beginning it is best to abstain altogether. Once the timing is appropriate, social media may be used but in extremely limited quantities. A time frame of 15 minutes is appropriate to avoid returning to a problem. Using a timer, social media limiting app, or someone to monitor your use is recommended at this point.

2. Stick to One App
   Limiting to one social media app rather than subscribing to many may also help here. If issues arise, then it is important to immediately abstain from social media use again.

3. Develop a Strong Support Network
   You should also build reinforcements. Having a support network including loved ones, family, friends, a therapist, and a support group is ideal. . . .

4. Have Healthy Off-Line Habits
   Participating in offline hobbies that promote health and wellness are ideal. Engaging in regular positive self-talk will increase self-esteem and reduce the need to receive attention through social media.

Matt Glowiak, "Social Media Addiction: Signs, Symptoms & Treatments," Choosing Therapy, February 23, 2022. www.choosingtherapy.com.

treatment, therapists and patients focus on the thoughts, or cognition, related to the addictive behavior, especially the thoughts that lead up to engaging in the behavior. When patients are able to pinpoint what they are thinking before opening an app or checking a screen, they can learn to react to those thoughts as they occur in real life, pause before acting on them, and avoid the addictive behavior.

Another effective treatment is known as dialectical behavior therapy (DBT). It is similar to CBT, but it adds mindfulness to the process of identifying thoughts and triggers for the addictive behavior. DBT helps patients pay attention not only to their thoughts but also to what is happening around them—what they see, hear, smell, and touch before engaging in the addictive behavior. Mindfulness helps DBT patients stay calm and avoid engaging in impulsive behavior.

Addressing Underlying Issues

Both CBT and DBT work by having patients focus on their conscious thoughts. Sometimes, however, the urge to engage with the virtual world may have roots in emotional issues simmering below the surface. The person might be going online to escape from or soothe anxiety or depression related to real-world problems, including physical abuse, sexual abuse, or an unhealthy family situation. "The commonality is that we are treating young people who are using screens to control the way they feel,"[68] says Michael Bishop, a psychologist who specializes in treating screen addiction. If the deep-seated feelings are not addressed, the treatment of the behavior alone will not succeed or, if it does, it might not last. In these cases, the person struggling with addiction needs to see a psychotherapist or psychiatrist. Since such sessions are not strictly limited to addiction therapy, their costs often will be covered by health insurance.

Sometimes, there are tensions within a family that are affecting all its members, and these family dynamics can be the underlying cause of screen addiction among its members. In such cases, the entire family may need to be treated together in a program known as family therapy. With this form of treatment, a therapist interviews family members together and separately to identify patterns

Residential Treatment Helps a Teen Out of Addiction

Dawn (not her real name) had a hard time making new friends when her family moved to a new state. To compensate, Dawn immersed herself in the digital world. Her parents tried to enforce limits on her screen time, but Dawn resisted. She fought with her parents and eventually started harming herself. She received treatment for depression, but her parents believed that her screen addiction had to be treated as well. Eventually, they enrolled Dawn in an outdoor residential treatment program that focuses on helping teens with screen addiction. Dawn writes,

> I didn't realize I was becoming addicted. I felt like I needed to have a phone with me at all times. Isolating myself to watch TV made me forget about reality, and in the moment it was nice to get away. At the end of the (wilderness) [treatment] program I realized how much I was thankful for it. If I hadn't gone there, I'd be dead. . . .
>
> I know it's hard. I had to do it. But I'm glad I did. I have a future in store for me—a bright one. I came from the darkness—emotional, physical, mental, and spiritual—and now I'm making a life in the light.

Quoted in Jennifer Clopton, "Parents' Desperate Fight vs. Teen Screen Addiction," WebMD, April 10, 2019. www.webmd.com.

of behavior that may be causing stress, anxiety, and dysfunction. Sometimes family behavior is being shaped by a root cause, such as a family member's substance abuse, a medical problem, or a death in the family. Once the therapist identifies the sources of the negative patterns, the family adopts a plan to address the problems as a group. The counselor continues to meet with the family to ensure communication is flowing and everyone is contributing to the needed changes. The screen addiction is treated along with all the other contributing factors until it is resolved.

In many cases, the person struggling with addiction may have an accompanying disorder, such as attention-deficit/hyperactivity disorder, substance abuse, anxiety, depression, or another disorder. Since the screen addiction and the disorder are linked, the patient needs a treatment that addresses both problems. This is known as dual diagnosis treatment. "Treat the problem," says addiction expert Maia Szalavitz. "You may need to deal with the screen in treating other issues, but if a kid is being bullied and spending a lot of time on screens, address the bullying. If a kid is anxious or depressed, treat that."[69]

Inpatient Treatment

Most individual treatment and family therapy is conducted on an outpatient basis. That is, the patients live at home while receiving treatment at a therapist's office for a certain number of hours a week. In extreme cases, however, outpatient treatment does not reduce or eliminate the addictive behavior. Patients may need to separate themselves from the home, school, or work and focus solely on overcoming their addiction at a live-in facility dedicated to treatment. Such facilities are known as residential treatment programs.

A patient usually is not alone at a residential treatment facility. Instead, the patient joins other people who are also struggling with addiction. Being surrounded by people facing the same problem often makes the patient feel understood and less isolated. In addition, the patient receives counseling, often as part of the group.

Twelve-Step Programs

Many residential treatment facilities treat addiction using a twelve-step program. First designed to treat alcoholism, twelve-step programs are now used to address a wide range of addictions—from gambling to overeating. As the name suggests, participants in twelve-step programs follow twelve time-tested steps to deal with the various aspects of addiction.

Twelve-step programs use a peer-to-peer model of treatment, with the addicted person meeting with a group of people who share the same addiction. No one else is allowed to participate in the treatment sessions, and everyone agrees that whatever is said in the meetings will remain private. Members go by their first names only, ensuring anonymity. With such safeguards in place, participants can be completely honest about their behavior without worrying that the information will be used against them outside the

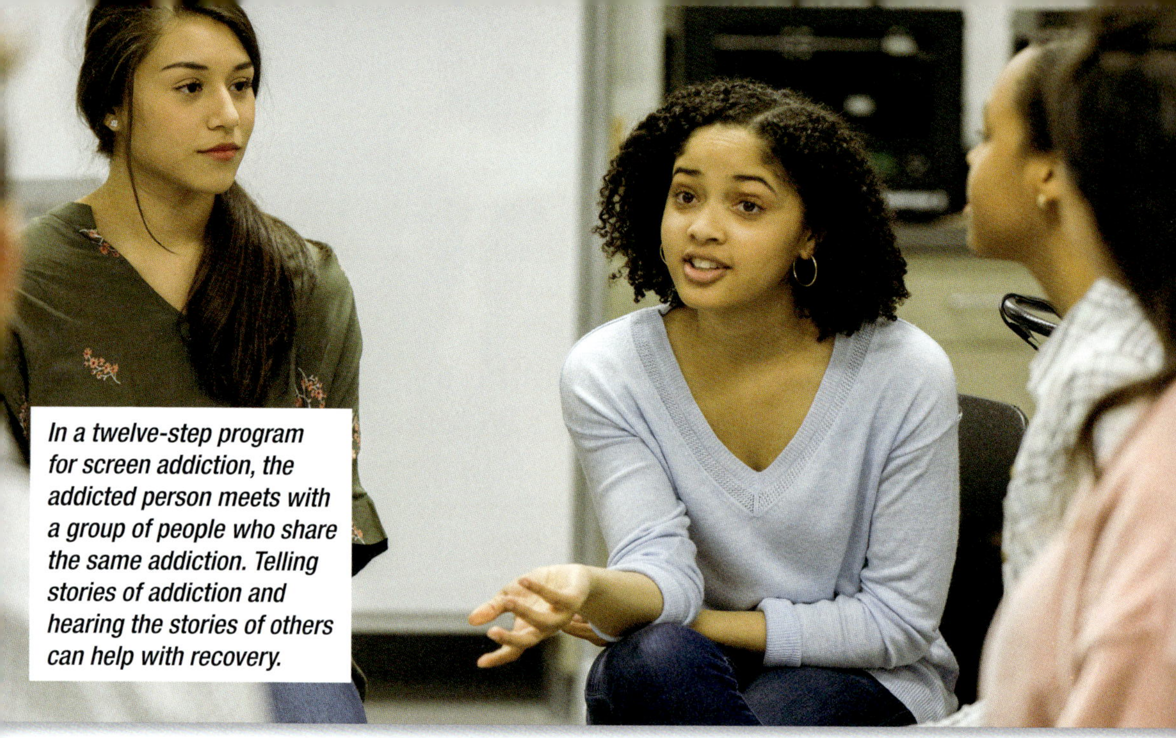

In a twelve-step program for screen addiction, the addicted person meets with a group of people who share the same addiction. Telling stories of addiction and hearing the stories of others can help with recovery.

group. By telling their stories of addiction, and hearing the stories of others, members of a twelve-step program receive acceptance, support, and guidance for overcoming their addiction.

No two people are alike, and no two screen addictions are the same, either. Some grow out of a fascination with streaming content. Others evolve from game play. And still others result from overexposure to social media. Some people have underlying mental conditions, family tensions, or substance abuse issues that contribute to their addiction. Others simply get hooked on the pleasures of the brain's own reward system. For some, many factors work together to overwhelm their ability to control their screen usage. Accordingly, the affected individuals must follow their own path out of addiction. Some can do it alone. Some do it with the assistance of technologies designed to support recovery. Others require professional help in its many forms. In extreme cases, only removal from the distractions of everyday life will enable these individuals to break the pattern of the addiction. Whatever the program or technique they use, recovering addicts will emerge with a renewed appreciation for the beauty of the real world and the people in it.

Introduction: A Growing Crisis

1. Lev, comment on Michael D. Pollock, "How I Overcame TV Addiction, Reclaimed My Life and Gained Two Months Per Year," February 9, 2020. www.michaeldpollock.com.
2. Vivek H. Murthy, *Protecting Youth Mental Health: The U.S. Surgeon General's Advisory*. Washington, DC: Office of the Surgeon General, US Department of Health and Human Services, 2021, p. 25. www.hhs.gov/sites/default/files/surgeon-general-youth-mental-health-advisory.pdf.

Chapter One: The Fear of Missing Out

3. Moya Lothian-McLean, "My Beautiful Dark Twisted Phone-Tasy: 10 Long Years of Phone Addiction," *gal-dem,* March 5, 2021. https://gal-dem.com.
4. Quoted in Trustmary, "7 Real Examples You Can Copy of Using Fear of Missing Out (FOMO) in Advertising," February 23, 2022. https://trustmary.com.
5. Quoted in Megan Teske, "Iowa State Research Shows That Some May Be at More Risk for Video Game Addiction," Iowa State Daily, November 6, 2018. www.iowastatedaily.com.
6. Quoted in Health Matters, "Is Social Media Threatening Teens' Mental Health and Well-Being?," February 28, 2020. https://healthmatters.nyp.org.
7. Victoria Rideout et al., *Coping with COVID-19: How Young People Use Digital Media to Manage Their Mental Health*. San Francisco: Common Sense and Hopelab, 2021, p. 10.
8. Quoted in Georgia Wells, Jeff Horwitz, and Deepa Seetharaman, "Facebook Knows Instagram Is Toxic for Teen Girls, Company Documents Show," *Wall Street Journal*, September 14, 2021. www.wsj.com.
9. Noor Bloemen and David De Coninck, "Social Media and Fear of Missing Out in Adolescents: The Role of Family Characteristics," *Social Media + Society*, October 21, 2020. https://journals.sagepub.com.
10. Bloemen and De Coninck, "Social Media and Fear of Missing Out in Adolescents."
11. Bloemen and De Coninck, "Social Media and Fear of Missing Out in Adolescents."

12. Sam Madden et al., *The Harsh Realities of Phone Distraction*. Cambridge, MA: Cambridge Mobile Telematics, 2020, p. 15.
13. Madden et al., *The Harsh Realities of Phone Distraction*, p. 17.
14. Quoted in Tanya Mohn, "'Troubling' Surge in Walker Deaths Despite Drop in Driving," *Forbes*, April 1, 2021. www.forbes.com.
15. Quoted in Camila Domonoske, "Pedestrian Fatalities Remain at 25-Year High for Second Year in a Row," *The Two-Way* (blog), National Public Radio, February 28, 2018. www.npr.org.
16. Tracey Folly, "Why I Deleted My Social Media Accounts," Medium, February 20, 2020. https://medium.com.
17. Quoted in *New Zealand Herald*, "Girl Suffers Fatal Electric Shock After Cellphone Falls in Bath," December 4, 2021. www.nzherald .co.nz.

Chapter Two: The Risks of Social Media

18. Quoted in Wells, Horwitz, and Seetharaman, "Facebook Knows Instagram Is Toxic for Teen Girls, Company Documents Show."
19. Quoted in Jean Twenge, "The Facebook Exposé: Four Things Parents Need to Know," Institute for Family Studies blog, October 11, 2021. https://ifstudies.org.
20. Quoted in Kate Linebaugh, "The Facebook Files, Part 6: The Whistleblower," *The Journal* (podcast), *Wall Street Journal*, October 3, 2021. www.wsj.com.
21. Quoted in Kari Paul, "Facebook Whistleblower Hearing: Frances Haugen Calls for More Regulation of Tech Giant," *The Guardian*, October 5, 2021. www.theguardian.com.
22. Quoted in Scott Pelley, "Whistleblower: Facebook Is Misleading the Public on Progress Against Hate Speech, Violence, Misinformation," CBS News, October 4, 2021. www.cbsnews.com.
23. Quoted in Wells, Horwitz, and Seetharaman, "Facebook Knows Instagram Is Toxic for Teen Girls, Company Documents Show."
24. Quoted in Kate Linebaugh, "The Facebook Files, Part 2: 'We Make Body Image Issues Worse,'" *The Journal* (podcast), *Wall Street Journal*, September 14, 2021. www.wsj.com.
25. Quoted in Linebaugh, "The Facebook Files, Part 2."
26. Quoted in Linebaugh, "The Facebook Files, Part 2."
27. Quoted in Wells, Horwitz, and Seetharaman, "Facebook Knows Instagram Is Toxic for Teen Girls, Company Documents Show."
28. Quoted in Wells, Horwitz, and Seetharaman, "Facebook Knows Instagram Is Toxic for Teen Girls, Company Documents Show."
29. Quoted in Pelley, "Whistleblower."
30. Quoted in Paul, "Facebook Whistleblower Hearing."

31. Quoted in Kevin T. Dugan, "What Facebook Is Hiding from Us," *Fortune*, September 14, 2021. https://fortune.com.
32. Twenge, "The Facebook Exposé."
33. Jean M. Twenge and W. Keith Campbell, "Associations Between Screen Time and Lower Psychological Well-Being Among Children and Adolescents: Evidence from a Population-Based Study," *Preventive Medicine Reports*, December 2018. www.ncbi.nlm.nih.gov.
34. Jean M. Twenge et al., "Specification Curve Analysis Shows That Social Media Use Is Linked to Poor Mental Health, Especially Among Girls," *Acta Psychologica*, April 2022. www.sciencedirect.com.

Chapter Three: The Lure of Online Gaming

35. Jack, "Gaming Got in the Way of What I Really Loved," Game Quitters (blog), November 11, 2019. https://gamequitters.com.
36. Jack, "Gaming Got in the Way of What I Really Loved."
37. Jack, "Gaming Got in the Way of What I Really Loved."
38. Andrew K. Przybylski, Netta Weinstein, and Kou Murayama, "Internet Gaming Disorder: Investigating the Clinical Relevance of a New Phenomenon," *American Journal of Psychiatry*, March 2017. https://ajp.psychiatryonline.org.
39. Przybylski, Weinstein, and Murayama, "Internet Gaming Disorder."
40. Douglas A. Gentile et al., "Internet Gaming Disorder in Children and Adolescents," *Pediatrics*, November 2017. https://pediatrics.aap publications.org.
41. Przybylski. Weinstein, and Murayama, "Internet Gaming Disorder."
42. Przybylski. Weinstein, and Murayama, "Internet Gaming Disorder."
43. Tom, "Gaming Made Me Destroy My Brother's Xbox," Game Quitters (blog), May 29, 2021. https://gamequitters.com.
44. Tom, "Gaming Made Me Destroy My Brother's Xbox."
45. Tom, "Gaming Made Me Destroy My Brother's Xbox."
46. Tom, "Gaming Made Me Destroy My Brother's Xbox."
47. Tom, "Gaming Made Me Destroy My Brother's Xbox."
48. Tom, "Gaming Made Me Destroy My Brother's Xbox."
49. Tom, "Gaming Made Me Destroy My Brother's Xbox."
50. Quoted in Marley Ghizzone, "Q&A: Gaming Addiction: The Newest Mental Health Disorder," *Infectious Diseases in Children*, July 10, 2018. www.healio.com.

Chapter Four: Designed to Engage

51. Quoted in Hilary Andersson, "Social Media Apps Are 'Deliberately' Addictive to Users," BBC News, July 4, 2018. www.bbc.com.

52. Quoted in Andersson, "Social Media Apps Are 'Deliberately' Addictive to Users."

53. Rebecca Fishbein, "How to Kick a Mindless Scrolling Habit," *Forge*, August 12, 2019. https://forge.medium.com.

54. Quoted in Fishbein, "How to Kick a Mindless Scrolling Habit."

55. Quoted in Andersson, "Social Media Apps Are 'Deliberately' Addictive to Users."

56. Quoted in Andersson, "Social Media Apps Are 'Deliberately' Addictive to Users."

57. Quoted in Mia Levitin, "The Like Button," Tortoise, April 5, 2021. www.tortoisemedia.com.

58. Quoted in Fishbein, "How to Kick a Mindless Scrolling Habit."

59. Quoted in Mattha Busby, "Social Media Copies Gambling Methods 'to Create Psychological Cravings,'" *The Guardian*, May 8, 2018. www.theguardian.com.

60. Quoted in Erin Bunch, "You Can Officially Hide Likes on Instagram—Here's Why Psychologists Say That's Good for Mental Health," Well + Good, April 28, 2021. www.wellandgood.com.

61. Quoted in Bunch, "You Can Officially Hide Likes on Instagram."

62. Quoted in BBC News, "Loot Boxes Linked to Problem Gambling in New Research," April 2, 2021. www.bbc.com.

63. Quoted in BBC News, "Loot Boxes Linked to Problem Gambling in New Research."

Chapter Five: Overcoming Screen Addiction

64. Arthur C. Brooks, "How to Break a Phone Addiction," *The Atlantic*, October 7, 2021. www.theatlantic.com.

65. Brooks, "How to Break a Phone Addiction."

66. Jack, "Gaming Got in the Way of What I Really Loved."

67. Jack, "Gaming Got in the Way of What I Really Loved."

68. Quoted in Jennifer Clopton, "Parents' Desperate Fight vs. Teen Screen Addiction," WebMD, April 10, 2019. www.webmd.com.

69. Quoted in Clopton, "Parents' Desperate Fight vs. Teen Screen Addiction."

Center for Humane Technology

www.humanetech.com

The Center for Humane Technology is a nonprofit organization dedicated to exposing the negative effects of social media and empowering people to break free from persuasive technology. The website includes a youth toolkit with seven self-guided lessons to help young people navigate the social media environment.

Computer Gaming Addicts Anonymous (CGAA)

www.cgaa.info

The CGAA offers a twelve-step program to help addicted gamers recover. The organization has seventy-one chapters in the United States and another ten around the world. In addition to face-to-face support groups, the CGAA offers online meetings, a discussion forum, and a help line. Its website provides an online test for video game addiction and stories of gaming addiction on YouTube.

Game Quitters

https://gamequitters.com

Game Quitters is an online community for gamers who want to stop playing video games. Its website offers an online quiz for gamers to assess how serious a problem they may have and a step-by-step guide to help them quit playing. It also provides a separate guide for family members and friends of gaming addicts to help them recognize and stop video game addiction. The website also provides a forum, personal stories, videos, and more.

Internet and Technology Addicts Anonymous (ITAA)

https://internetaddictsanonymous.org

ITAA offers twelve-step treatment through online and face-to-face meetings for a variety of screen addictions, including internet and technology addiction, streaming addiction, social media addiction, and smartphone addiction. The website offers tools for recovery and a list of meeting locations.

MediaSmarts

https://mediasmarts.ca

MediaSmarts is a Canadian not-for-profit charitable organization dedicated to teaching digital and media literacy. It promotes critical thinking skills so that children and youth can engage with media as active and informed digital citizens.

reSTART Life

www.netaddictionrecovery.com

The organization offers both outpatient and inpatient treatment programs that specialize in problematic internet, video game, and technology use. It works with individuals, couples, and families to better understand and address addiction and to create an individualized plan to promote a healthy, balanced lifestyle.

FOR FURTHER RESEARCH

Books

Adam Alter, *Irresistible: The Rise of Addictive Technology and the Business of Keeping Us Hooked*. New York: Penguin, 2018.

Mark Carrier, *From Smartphones to Social Media: How Technology Affects Our Brains and Behavior.* Santa Barbara, CA: Greenwood, 2018.

Jaron Lanier, *Ten Arguments for Deleting Your Social Media Accounts Right Now*. New York: Henry Holt, 2018.

Bradley Steffens, *Cell Phone Addiction*. San Diego: ReferencePoint, 2020.

Marysia Weber, *Screen Addiction: Why You Can't Put That Phone Down*. St. Louis: En Route Books & Media, 2019.

Internet Sources

Tracey Folly, "Why I Deleted My Social Media Accounts," Medium, February 20, 2020. https://medium.com.

Kate Linebaugh, "The Facebook Files, Part 2: 'We Make Body Image Issues Worse,'" *The Journal* (podcast), *Wall Street Journal*, September 14, 2021. www.wsj.com.

Moya Lothian-McLean, "My Beautiful Dark Twisted Phone-Tasy: 10 Long Years of Phone Addiction," *gal-dem*, March 5, 2021. https://gal-dem.com.

Gigen Mammoser, "The FOMO Is Real: How Social Media Increases Depression and Loneliness," Healthline, December 9, 2018. www.healthline.com.

The Dorm, "Treating 'Screen Addiction' in Young Adults," April 6, 2019. https://thedorm.com.

Jean Twenge, "The Facebook Exposé: Four Things Parents Need to Know," Institute for Family Studies blog, October 11, 2021. https://ifstudies.org.

INDEX